# Intermittent Fasting

*Burn Fat And Build Muscle Through Intermittent Fasting For Rapid Weight Loss and a Healthier Lifestyle for Men and Women*

*Elliot Cutting*

# Table of Contents

**Introduction to Intermittent Fasting**

It's Easy to Lose Fat with Intermittent Fasting

*1. Calories*

*2. Therapeutic*

*3. Autophagy*

What Are the Origins of Fasting?

Reasons Why People Fast

Why is Intermittent Fasting the Easiest Approach?

What makes Intermittent Fasting different from Other Weight Loss Programs?

It is a Diet of Foodies

What Are Doctors Saying About Intermittent Fasting?

Calorie intake is crucial

**Chapter 1: Intermittent Fasting Lifestyle**

How to Begin the Transition

Getting Started with Intermittent Fasting

5 Common Mistakes People Make when Transitioning to Intermittent Fasting

Eat your Favorite Foods and Still Lose Weight

Self-Discipline and Intermittent Fasting

**Chapter 2: Types of Fasting**

1. The 16/8 Fasting Protocol

*Positive attributes of the 16/8 fasting protocol*

*Things to Keep in Mind*

2. The 5-2 Fast Diet Protocol

   *500 – 600 Calories*

   *5-2 Protocol for Weight Loss*

   *Eating on Your Fast Days*

3. Alternate-Day Fasting

4. The 24-Hour Fast Protocol

Spontaneous and Convenient Meal Skipping

The 16/8 Protocol is Highly Recommended

**Chapter 3: Transitioning to Intermittent Fasting**

  Getting Started with Intermittent Fasting

   *Additional steps to get you started*

   *Other Crucial Considerations*

   *Now Begin the Transition*

**Chapter 4: Counting Your Calorie Intake**

  What are Macronutrients?

  Counting Macronutrients

   *Tracking macros*

   *How to Track Macronutrients*

   *Calculating Macros for Weight Loss*

  Best Time to Work Out when Fasting

**Chapter 5: Health Benefits of Intermittent Fasting**

  Evidence-Based Benefits of Intermittent Fasting

  Health Benefits of Calorie Restrictions

  Advice and Tips for Successful Intermittent Fasting

**Chapter 6: Food Guide**

  Food and Nutrition

*Nutrient-Dense Foods*

*Include Probiotics in Your Diet*

*Foods to Avoid*

*Best Foods to Eat on Intermittent Fasting*

*Tips about Food, Meals, and Nutrition*

*Intermittent Fasting and Alcohol*

**Chapter 7: Getting Started with Intermittent Fasting**

Reorganize your meals

*The One Week Kick-Start Plan*

*Actions for Insane and Rapid Weight Loss*

**Chapter 8: Maintaining the Fast**

Make Intermittent Fasting Work for You

Why You Should Stick with Intermittent Fasting Long-Term

How to Handle Initial Fasting Challenges

How to Make Intermittent Fasting Easy on the Body

Tracking Progress and Keeping Motivated

**Chapter 9: Diseases Treated or Cured**

**Chapter 10: Myths, Common Questions, and Considerations for Men and Women**

Breakfast Myths

10 Popular Questions on Intermittent Fasting

Men and Intermittent Fasting – Things to Consider

Women and Intermittent Fasting – Things to Consider

**Chapter 11: Popular Intermittent Fasting Celebrities**

**Conclusion**

# Introduction to Intermittent Fasting

Intermittent fasting is a term that refers to a healthy lifestyle trend that is gaining popularity around the world. It involves alternate cycles of eating and fasting. In very simple terms, intermittent fasting involves making a conscious decision to skip one or two meals deliberately.

Dieters follow this lifestyle because of its numerous, proven benefits. These benefits include improved metabolic health, weight loss, longevity, protection against diseases, and a healthy body.

Intermittent fasting is more than just fasting. It is a lifestyle that requires you to take in calories at certain specific times of the day and then consuming absolutely nothing for the remainder of the day.

## It's Easy to Lose Fat with Intermittent Fasting

There are plenty of diets out there that people follow. However, more and more health-conscious individuals are choosing intermittent fasting because it works, it is backed by science, it is manageable for the long term, and has numerous health benefits.

### 1. Calories

A lot of people have misconstrued ideas about why we put on weight. They think it is the choice of food or lack of physical activity. However, according to science, we put on weight because of the consumption of excess calories. Excessive calorie intake is the reason why we put on weight.

By deliberately skipping meals, we reduce our caloric intake on a regular basis. When we reduce the amount of food we eat, then we automatically lose weight. This is the main principle behind intermittent fasting lifestyle and this is why you are still able to eat your favorite foods because your eating window is shortened.

## 2. Therapeutic

For many centuries, doctors have acknowledged the healing powers of fasting. Since the early 1900s, doctors have successfully used intermittent fasting to address health problems such as diabetes, epilepsy, and obesity.

This approach is now making a successful comeback. Intermittent fasting is now common. Dieters prefer this lifestyle because of its health, weight loss, and therapeutic benefits. By fasting, you get all these healing and therapeutic benefits.

## 3. Autophagy

One of the most powerful benefits of intermittent fasting is brought about by autophagy. Autophagy is the body's ultimate recycling system. Now, whenever we fast, we set into motion the process of autophagy. When cells in our bodies are deprived of calories, they initiate this process.

Autophagy replaces worn-out and damaged parts of your cells with new ones. This helps to preserve tissue health. Cells in your body create a membrane that hunts down worn-out, diseased, and dead cells and then consumed them. The resulting molecule is then used to create new cell components and to produce energy. In the process, cells also get rid of toxins and consume harmful organism such as those that cause diseases.

Therefore, autophagy performs an effective detoxification throughout the body, helping to eliminate harmful, disease-causing pathogens, eliminating diseased and worn out cells and also reducing inflammation. Normally, autophagy happens when cells in the body digest proteins in order to release amino acids to produce much-needed energy in the body. This process slows down the aging process and promotes metabolism.

# What Are the Origins of Fasting?

Fasting simply means deliberate abstinence from drink, food, or both for a specific period of time. It comes in different forms depending on where you live. Absolute fasting is one type. This type of fasting requires total abstinence from all food and drink for a period of about 24 hours.

Man has been fasting for various reasons since time immemorial. Humans and animals naturally resort to fasting during sickness or moments of high stress. Fasting is crucial because it provides rest, balance, and also for energy conservation at critical moments.

Early philosophers, healers, great thinkers, mathematicians, and physicists used fasting as a therapy for healing purposes. Some of these intellectuals include Socrates, Aristotle, Hippocrates, Galen, and Plato. They all spoke favorably about fasting and how therapeutic it is.

Fasting is also common among nearly all major religions of the world. These include Buddhism, Islam, Judaism, and Christianity. Fasting for religious purposes is common among these religions. Faithful fast in order to appeal to a higher deity and sometimes as a form of sacrifice and even cleansing.

Other people and communities fast as part of their traditions. For instance, the Indians of both north and South America fast regularly as they observe certain traditions such as praying for rain or mourning the passing of a great person. Healers of the 19th century used fasting as a form of healing therapy. Yoga practice, which has some fasting elements, has been around for thousands of years. Even ancient healing practices such as Ayurveda include some forms of fasting. Even ordinary people such as you and I practice overnight fasting just about every single day.

# Reasons Why People Fast

For religious reasons
Political reasons
Health reasons – to treat an ailment
Medical reasons – for medical procedures, diagnostic purposes

# Why is Intermittent Fasting the Easiest Approach?

Research has shown that intermittent fasting is extremely effective when it comes to weight loss – and especially fat loss. It is just as effective as calorie restriction but easier especially compared to other types of diets because of a number of reasons.

## 1. Intermittent fasting causes insulin levels to drop

When we eat, insulin levels in the body increase. This makes it difficult to lose weight. However, when we fast, insulin levels fall significantly. This allows the body to access fat reserves for energy.

Numerous studies have confirmed that intermittent fasting will not only help to reduce weight but also improve body composition even though results may vary from individual to individual. A study in the 2017 issue of JAMA Internal Medicine shows that dieters stand to lose between 5% and 6% of total body weight when they tried intermittent fasting.

## 2. Intermittent fasting helps you to retain lean muscle

One of the benefits of losing weight through intermittent fasting is that you only lose fat and not muscle. This is according to Krista Varady, Ph.D., a research scientist at the University of Illinois in Chicago. She is also an associate professor of nutrition and kinesiology at the same institution.

According to her findings, most people who lose weight typically lose 75% fat and 25% muscle mass. However, with intermittent fasting, over 90% of weight loss is fat.

### 3. You are able to control cravings

One of the reasons why we put on so much weight is because we succumb to cravings. We crave sugar and starch because our bodies are so used to them. Fortunately, when you adopt an intermittent fasting lifestyle, all your cravings will eventually disappear. You will no longer have cravings for unhealthy foods and snacks anymore.

### 4. Intermittent fasting will drastically reduce cholesterol and triglyceride levels

According to studies recorded in Nutrition Reviews, intermittent fasting has been shown to reduce not just body fat but also triglycerides and cholesterol levels. This is in both overweight and normal weight individuals. This mostly has to do with insulin levels. When you consume fewer calories each day, your blood sugar levels will come down and insulin levels will stabilize.

### Is there a catch?

Intermittent fasting is so effective when it comes to weight loss that some people wonder if there is a catch or downside. However, experts agree that there is no real downside to this lifestyle. It is a pretty safe approach to how you eat and live and hardly ever leads to eating disorders.

The only minor challenge that most dieters experience is at the beginning when they have to battle hunger. You can expect the first five days to be challenging because you will feel hungry. However, there are ways to combat hunger pangs. If you are busy, then you mind will most likely not focus on the hunger but on other things.

# What makes Intermittent Fasting different from Other Weight Loss Programs?

There are many reasons why intermittent fasting is much better and more effective compared to other diets and weight loss programs. The single most important factor is that intermittent fasting is a lifestyle and not a diet.

Intermittent fasting is a lifestyle that requires you to consciously skip meals occasionally. Most other diets are temporary and have unrealistic goals and requirements. Some are dangerous because of what they require of you. However, intermittent fasting has been proven by health experts, researchers, and others to be effective and manageable in the long run.

Intermittent fasting does not dictate what foods you should eat. What it does is dictate when you should eat and when you should fast. However, to gain the most benefits from this lifestyle, it is advisable to eat natural foods, healthy meals, and nutrients from all major food groups. This way, your body will receive all the essential nutrition it requires from the various food groups.

You can expect to live your best life free from major illnesses and chronic conditions. Since intermittent fasting advocates for a physically active lifestyle, you will enjoy an all-around healthy lifestyle. It also promotes longevity based on numerous studies that have been published.

## It is a Diet of Foodies

Sometimes intermittent fasting is referred to as a diet for foodies. A foodie is simply any person who has a keen interest and finer taste for food. Most foodies have gone through a number of diets and the results have not always been pleasant.

If you follow this diet or lifestyle, you will not be limited by food choice. Intermittent fasting actually offers the ultimate flexibility when it comes to food choice. This implies that you are free to enjoy a wide variety of foods even those that are forbidden by other diets and you will still benefit from regular fasts. You will still have to watch your calories but having such a wide variety of foods to choose from is definitely liberating and this makes this lifestyle stand out from the rest.

## What Are Doctors Saying About Intermittent Fasting?

Doctors have heard about all the numerous diets and eating patterns out there. They have also read on some of the popular ones like intermittent fasting. However, only intermittent fasting is backed by research and evidence. Most health professionals are impressed with the research findings.

One of the most recent studies, about Cell Metabolism, showcases the benefits of intermittent fasting. The study shows that cutting calories even for short periods of time can bring about serious changes to your body and overall health. However, you should speak to your doctor to ensure that you eat right and do not lose out on important nutrients, especially on fasting days.

Doctors believe this is an excellent lifestyle that, if followed correctly, then it can lead to a healthy lifestyle, weight loss and so much more. Doctors believe that sufficient precaution should be taken. For instance, dieters should not fast for extended periods of time and they should not have any health concerns.

For instance, someone with certain health conditions should generally refrain from partaking in this diet unless with advice from a physician. For instance, pregnant and lactating women, anyone with a history of eating disorders, and those recovering from surgery should refrain from this lifestyle.

# Calorie intake is crucial

From the research findings, a lot of the doctors believe it all has to do with calorie intake. The reason is that most dieters who follow this lifestyle follow other diets such as ketogenic, Mediterranean, and so on. When calorie intake is limited, then even overweight and obese individuals will lose weight. Losing weight comes with other benefits such as stable insulin levels, lower blood pressure, better metabolic rate, and also lower cardiovascular risk.

Such a lifestyle should be adapted for the long-term and should not be treated as a fad diet for short-term gain. Diet should not be reduced to an unhealthy cycle of binge eating and calorie restriction because this will defeat the intended purpose. Discipline is necessary and having goals in mind is crucial for long-term success.

Rather than let this lifestyle define you, you should instead focus on good health and getting proper nourishment. When you eat clean, you become healthier and will avoid chronic conditions like heart disease and high blood pressure. Make sure you increase your fruit and vegetable consumption and reduce your carbs intake. If you find a plan that works for you, then you will become mentally and physically healthy and happy.

# Chapter 1: Intermittent Fasting Lifestyle

Intermittent fasting lifestyle requires you to adjust your eating habits. When you start following this lifestyle religiously, you will have to deny your body food for a number of hours on particular days.

Intermittent fasting is a lifestyle rather than a diet. You will, therefore, need to be very clear about what you are getting yourself into. Food is usually a big deal in most cultures and our lives revolve around it. As a dieter, you should know that intermittent fasting consists of a number of different protocols. These protocols define fasting and eating times. For instance, we have protocols such as the 5-2 and the 8-6.

The 5-2 protocol dictates normal eating for five days of the week followed by fasting for 2 days of the week. You need to find the intermittent fasting protocol that works for you and suits your regular schedules. For instance, if you are a morning person, then choose a protocol that goes well with mornings.

Also, when choosing your preferred fasting protocol, you should think about the reasons why you are fasting and your regular schedules. Some people are extremely busy during the week but only slightly busy on the weekends. Others wish to lose weight. What you need to do is to ensure that your preferred fasting protocol is in tandem with your lifestyle.

## How to Begin the Transition

The transition part is probably going to be your most challenging part. This is because you will start to fast on a regular basis. Your main focus at this time should be to ease into your preferred protocol. You can, for instance, delay your next meal by a couple of hours. If you are in the habit of snacking at midnight, try and cut this out because it is not healthy.

While this lifestyle is majorly about fasting and easing, its success is based on your mental situation. You should train your mind to adjust to this lifestyle. You can, for instance, delay your breakfast by about an hour and then stop your evening meals an hour earlier than usual in order to train the mind of the impending lifestyle changes.

This kind of training of the mind is akin to the way muscles are trained. You first begin training with a lightweight and gradually proceed to increase your weight. This process will continue as you gradually modify your eating habits and general lifestyle.

# Getting Started with Intermittent Fasting

One of the main requirements of intermittent fasting is that you change your eating habits. This lifestyle does not necessarily deprive you of food but rather it dictates when you eat and when you fast. Once you begin this lifestyle, then you will have to learn how to go for long stretches without eating.

In most cultures around the world, food is a huge aspect of life and our lives kind of revolve around it. It is crucial that you select the most appropriate protocol so that this new lifestyle works for you. Here are some of the best ways to get started.

o *Choose your preferred fasting protocol*

There are different kinds of protocols that you can follow. They include the 5-2, 16/8, eat-stop-eat, and so on. Think about your lifestyle such as work schedule, family commitments, exercise times, and so on. Find the protocol that best suits your lifestyle.

There are also other factors that you should consider. For instance, what are your reasons for fasting? Most people fast in order to lose weight. If your aim is to lose lots of weight, then you may want to consider the eat-stop-eat or the modified version of the 16-8 protocol where you fast for 18 hours with an eating window of only 6 hours.

   o   *Adjust your eating habits*

Plenty of people who start the intermittent fasting lifestyle often consume unhealthy food options. They eat plenty of junk food, processed food, carbonated drinks and so on. The problem with unhealthy eating habits is that they affect your blood sugar, moods, energy levels, and hormones.

You should adjust your diet and start eating clean. Go for healthy, natural foods like vegetables and fruits, whole grains, juices, salads, nuts, and seeds. A healthier diet and regular workouts will result in a healthy body and long-term weight loss.

# 5 Common Mistakes People Make when Transitioning to Intermittent Fasting

### 1. Fear of being hungry even for a little while
Feeling hungry is part of life and happens to all of us. In fact, we are hungry a lot of the time. However, being hungry for a couple of hours is generally okay. The hunger pangs will not kill you neither will your strong and lean muscles disappear. This is a fact that has been proven over and over again.

You can lose weight and keep it off while at the same time working out at the gym. Health and fitness expert Jeremy Scott has personal experience when it comes to intermittent fasting. He advises dieters to stick to this lifestyle while lifting weights and generally working out on a regular basis. This way, you will be able to develop lean and strong muscles.

Also, being hungry for a couple of hours will not kill you. Your digestive system will actually benefit from the break. It is very possible to go even 16 to 18 to 24 hours in office. Short-term fasting such as the protocols of intermittent fasting will not cause any significant muscle damage. There are numerous studies that claim that this is actually the case.

## 2. Eating junk food most of the time

You will not be successful in the long run if you keep eating junk foods, processed foods, fizzy drinks and all that. Experts say that you cannot build a million dollar home on a $1 salary. This statement is absolutely correct.

One of the most common phrases people say is, "I struggle with fat loss." However, you will find that most of the time it has to do with nutrition. Most of the time people do not eat right.

Any person who is struggling with weight loss after adopting the intermittent fasting lifestyle is probably eating the wrong kind of food. Poor quality meals and snacks make it hard to lose weight. Remember that limiting your calorie intake is the best solution to losing weight and keeping it off.

So you need to watch your calorie intake and also ensure that you eat quality calories all the time. This means eating mostly fresh natural foods like fruits and vegetables and avoiding processed foods as much as possible.

## 3. Jumping into intermittent fasting too fast

One of the reasons why people fail at lifestyle changes and diets is because of jumping in too fast. It is advisable to take a moment and appreciate that intermittent fasting lifestyle is probably completely different from what we are used to.

For instance, if you are used to eating or snacking every two hours and then jump into intermittent fasting, you will find it hard to keep up with the changes. It is advisable to begin slowly and follow protocols such as the 12-12 method. This protocol is ideal for beginners and allows you to fast for 12 hours and then

19

have your meals inside a 12-hour window. A lot of dieters start off this way and many stick to this particular protocol.

### 4. *You eat too much during your eating window*
Another very common mistake that beginners make is to eat too much during the eating window. While this lifestyle does not dictate what foods you should eat, common practice dictates that you limit your calorie intake to between 2200 calories for women and 2600 calories for men.

Even if you have been fasting for hours, you still need to watch what you eat. Consuming too many calories during your eating window will constitute excessive calories that will be stored in the body as fat. This will defeat the intended purpose of this otherwise beneficial lifestyle. Sometimes we get so physically and emotionally detached that when the time comes to eat, we overindulge. Therefore, try not to be too preoccupied with your next meal as this is a recipe for disaster.

### 5. *Being too ambitious*
Sometimes people start off with extremely high expectations. We notice a friend who has lost plenty of weight due to intermittent lifestyle and decide to jump right in. Some may expect to lose plenty of weight in just a few days. However, you should not be too hard on yourself and do not be too ambitious because the outcome may disappoint you.

Moving from six meals a day to only one meal a day is not only ambitious but rather extreme by any standards. Instead of taking such drastic steps, you should aim for steady but gradual steps until you get used to the new lifestyle. There are other protocols that you can pursue that are pretty effective. Think about the 16-8 protocol or the eat-stop-eat protocol. These are not very taxing and relatively easy to adapt. If you pursue this lifestyle, then you should do so in a structured manner.

# Eat your Favorite Foods and Still Lose Weight

Did you know that you can eat your favorite foods and still lose weight? With intermittent fasting, this is very possible. The reason is that intermittent fasting tells you when to eat but not what to eat. Basically, you are not denied your favorite foods. This lifestyle simply advises you when you should eat.

Most of us have a particular food or foods that we cherish. However, sometimes these favorite foods can keep us from losing weight and keeping it off. There are numerous diets out there that deprive us of our favorite foods. Even then, most of these diets do not work or are short-term in nature. Fortunately, intermittent fasting allows you to enjoy your favorite foods while losing weight and leading a healthy lifestyle.

During your fasting period, you should not consume any calories. However, you are allowed to drink water and calorie-free beverages such as black coffee and green tea. During your eating window, you can then have any meal that you like. However, you should watch your calories. This means consuming the recommended amount of calories in order to lose weight or maintain lean muscle. You are supposed to eat clean, healthy, and natural foods most of the time. Therefore if you love meats like steak, chicken, or fish, then you can have these but in moderation.

Intermittent fasting promotes the genes that burn fat and calories. Genes that uncouple proteins and enzymes that are crucial in fat oxidation are activated through fasting. Once these proteins are uncoupled, they produce holes in mitochondria within the body. The mitochondria will then produce less energy because of the holes.

Your body will then be forced to burn more calories in order to produce more energy. Therefore, fasting not only deprives your body of calories but also enhances caloric burn the whole day. When intermittent fasting is done correctly, you may end up eating most of your favorite foods and still lose weight and maintain muscle mass.

## Self-Discipline and Intermittent Fasting

If you really want to enjoy the benefits brought about by this lifestyle, then you need to be disciplined. Without discipline, then the lifestyle will probably not work out for you.

One of the most crucial steps is to focus on the benefits of this lifestyle. This will help to keep you motivated. When you feel motivated, then discipline will come automatically.

Discipline means not cheating during fasting. You should not consume any foods or snacks as you fast. Discipline also means avoiding foods that are not good for you such as processed foods, junk foods, and so on. Ensure that you do not consume excessive calories and only eat sufficient amounts of food.

You need to keep in mind that nothing is instant or easy and that everything takes time. Make sure that you keep your mind on your goals and let your desired goals keep you motivated. You should increase your food choice and eat a wide variety. Basically, the wider the variety the better it is for you.

# Chapter 2: Types of Fasting

Research findings released in 2017 have shown that intermittent fasting can provide benefits similar to those brought on by calorie restrictions. Calorie restriction has numerous benefits. For instance, it has been proven as the only experimental approach that extends lifespan by 30% and improves the prospects of patients with cancer. However, research has proven that intermittent fasting is more effective compared to calorie restriction.

Health experts such as doctors believe that fasting is actually an excellent idea. It is advisable to starve the body of nutrition a few hours each week a couple of times each week. There is plenty of evidence to showcase the benefits of managed food deprivation. There are different ways of depriving the body of calories. In intermittent fasting, these methods are known as protocols.

There are quite a number of intermittent protocols out there. The choice of protocol by dieters is really a matter of personal preference. There is no one protocol that is better than others. However, some could be more effective than others. You really should find one that fits perfectly with your lifestyle. Some of the common protocols include:

- o The 16/8 fasting protocol
- o The 5-2 protocol
- o Eat-sleep-eat protocol
- o The 24-hour fast
- o 18/6 fast protocol

The aim of each protocol is to advise you about when to fast and when to eat. However, the basic aim of each protocol is to allow you to fast for a period of time before eventually feasting on purpose. Let us examine these protocols in greater detail.

# 1. The 16/8 Fasting Protocol

One of the most popular ways of performing intermittent fasting is known as the 16-8 fasting protocols. This protocol requires you to fast for a total of 16 hours within a 24-hour period. You will then have all your meals within an 8-hour window.

As an example, you can have your last meal of the day at 8.00 pm in the night. You will then go to bed at 10.00 pm or 11.00 pm and have nothing to eat until 16 hours later or 12.00 noon the following day. You will then have all your meals and snacks within the next 8 hours or until 8.00 pm the following evening.

You can repeat this cycle as often as you want or follow it a couple of days per week depending on your preferences. This particular protocol has become very popular with dieters around the world especially those seeking to burn fat and lose weight.

While other diet fads and protocols often set out strict regulations and rules, the 16/8 protocol is very simple and easy to follow. It does not place any undue burden on dieters yet it delivers actual results with minimal effort. Apart from enhancing weight loss, this protocol enhances longevity, boosts brain function, and improves blood sugar control.

## Positive attributes of the 16/8 fasting protocol

Following this intermittent fasting protocol has been shown to be beneficial to the body in numerous ways all the way to cellular level. Here is a look at some of the benefits associated with this specific fasting protocol.

- o It causes insulin levels in the body to drop to very low levels. This helps the body to burn fat, optimize blood sugar levels and improve the body's insulin sensitivity

- It results in an increase in the body's levels of HGH or human growth hormone. HGH is a useful hormone that plays a huge role in decreasing body fat and improving the body's composition. The human growth hormone is also extremely useful in matters of cellular regeneration

- Intermittent fasting protocols such as the 16/8 have been shown to trigger important cellular repair processes like autophagy. Autophagy helps to repair old, worn out, and damaged cells as well as eliminate waste and keep the body healthy

When you follow this protocol, you will be able to fit in between two and four meals within the 8-hour eating window. The 16-8 protocol is also known as the Leangains protocol. You are able to make it a very simple fasting protocol by simply choosing not to have any snacks after dinner and then skipping breakfast the following morning.

Therefore, if your last meal was at 9.00 pm the previous evening, then ensure that you do not have any snacks for the rest of the evening and even the following morning. You will have your next meal the following day at 1.00 pm. You will by this time have fasted for 16 hours straight.

## Things to Keep in Mind

Always ensure that you eat mostly healthy foods such as fresh vegetables, lots of fruits, lean meat, whole grains, and so on. The 16/8 protocol is the easiest to follow and also the most natural way of following intermittent fasting. Even as you follow this protocol, ensure that you avoid junk foods and foods that are overly-processed as these are not good for your body.

# 2. The 5-2 Fast Diet Protocol

The other protocol that is popular with intermittent fasting is the 5–2 protocol which is also known as the fast diet. There are those who believe that this particular protocol is the most popular of all intermittent fasting protocols. One reason why it is so popular is because it allows you to eat normally for five days of the week and then you get to fast for only two days of the week.

The fasting days should be non-consecutive rather than consecutive. Therefore you will have to restrict your calorie intake for two non-consecutive by limiting your meals to a total of 500 – 600 calories per day.

A lot of dieters find this particular protocol easy to follow and easier to adapt compared to others. And since you do not have to fast each and every single day, this protocol is considered more of a lifestyle than a diet. It does not dictate any foods that you should or should not eat but only when to fast and when to eat.

## 500 – 600 Calories

During your fast days, you will consume a total of 500 calories for women and 600 calories for men. You will fast for most of the day and then only eat during your 8-hour eating window. For the remainder of the week, you are allowed to eat normally and have regular meals.

## 5-2 Protocol for Weight Loss

One of the benefits of this protocol is that it is effective for weight loss. If you follow it correctly, then you will lose weight and body fat. This is because this diet requires you to limit your calorie intake not just on your fasting days but even on days when you don't fast. It is important therefore that you do not over-indulge on your non-fast days.

If you follow this diet as recommended, then you should expect to lose between 3% and 8% of your body weight within 3 to 24 weeks. This is according to a study published here in this scientific journal. This study shows that properly abiding by the 5-2 protocol will help you lose anywhere between 4% and 8% of your waist circumference. This means losing large amounts of dangerous belly fat.

## Eating on Your Fast Days

There is generally no guiding rule on how to eat on your fast days. Some people prefer eating nothing all day and then have their meals during the small eating window. Others prefer having a small breakfast and then a meal much later in the evening. What you need to keep in mind is that you should eat a maximum of 500 calories for women and 600 calories for men. It is advisable, as such, to plan your meals accordingly. Ensure that your meals are healthy, full of fiber, and sufficient nutrition. High protein, low-glycemic carbs, vegetables, and fruits are highly recommended. These foods are not only highly nutritious but will also keep you feeling full for longer.

# 3. Alternate-Day Fasting

Another intermittent fasting protocol that is out there is the alternate-day protocol. This protocol requires you to fast every other day. This means you will alternate between fast days and normal eating days. You can modify this protocol to eat a maximum of 500 calories on your fast days and about 2200 – 2600 on non-fast days.

This particular protocol is very popular and effective for weight loss. It also comes with numerous other benefits. Your eating is only restricted half of the time but the benefits that you receive are immense. You can drink as much water and non-caloric beverages as you like. Non-caloric beverages include green tea, black coffee, and unsweetened tea. You should avoid all other types of drinks especially those sugary drinks, sodas, and carbonated drinks. These are not good for your body. This protocol allows you to consume between 20% and 25% of your energy requirements which totals to about 500 calories.

Studies done by nutrition scientists at the University of Chicago show that those who follow intermittent fasting can lose as much as 8% of their body weight in 3 to 12 weeks. This lifestyle is particularly useful for women as well especially those aged between 40 to 60 years. It helps to reduce stubborn belly fat and the results are far more impressive compared to traditional weight loss methods. Intermittent fasting is the number one choice for numerous dieters because it is easy to follow, has very few restrictions, is very effective and with amazing outcomes.

## 4. The 24-Hour Fast Protocol

Yet another method of following the intermittent fasting is the 24-hour protocol. This protocol requires you to fast for a 24-hour period or an entire day. For instance, if you have your last meal tonight at 8.00 pm, then you will eat nothing for the next 24 hours until 8.00 pm the following evening. However, you do not have to adhere to this protocol each and every day or even every other day. You can instead choose to apply it once or twice a week.

One reason why some prefer this protocol is because of issues to do with impulse eating or binge eating. People tend to eat when they feel lonely, excited, frustrated, happy, confused, or stressed. This means the food is used to address our emotional situation. Using food as a response to emotions does not provide the best approach to these issues. Feeding emotional hunger instead of real hunger is definitely not acceptable.

This particular fast enables you to differentiate between emotional and actual hunger. If you learn how to do without food even when stressed or emotional, then you will eventually learn how to cope with your emotions without then need for food.

In some cases, you may be unable to go without food for an entire 24-hour period. Fortunately, intermittent fasting is a flexible lifestyle that allows you to make acceptable adjustments. For instance, if you are unable to fast for an entire 24-hour period, then it is okay to fast for 22, 20, or even 18 hours. In short, you should not give up hope if things do not quite work out the first time. Just do the best that you can and keep improving on that.

## Spontaneous and Convenient Meal Skipping

Apart from the above protocols, there are other flexible forms of intermittent fasting that are widely accepted. Remember that the aim of this lifestyle is to go for long stretches of time without having anything to eat. One such protocol allows you to skip a meal whenever it is convenient to do so. There is no protocol to follow or rules to adhere with. All you simply do is skip a meal whenever possible and stand to see the results thereafter.

You can choose to skip a meal whenever you are busy or not feeling very hungry. There have been previous misconceptions about having to eat so many meals each day. However, this is not always the case and you can skip meals occasionally. You will suffer no harm if you skip a meal yet you stand to enjoy certain benefits.

The human body is aptly designed to handle stress including hunger. Meal skipping is not a stressful form of fasting but rather a convenient one that can be adapted from time to time. Even this simple approach has some health benefits to you so try and see where you fit best with these different fasting protocols.

## The 16/8 Protocol is Highly Recommended

If you want to adopt the intermittent fasting lifestyle, then you should opt for the 16/8 protocol. This is the model practiced successfully by most dieters. You are likely to succeed following this protocol compared to others especially if you wish to lose weight and keep it off. For long-term health and wellness, the 16/8 protocol offers you the best chance for success.

# Chapter 3: Transitioning to Intermittent Fasting

Intermittent fasting requires you to change your meal times so that you stay for lengthy periods of time without eating. This lifestyle offers you an excellent opportunity to lose body fat, weight, and maintain lean muscle. It will enable you to drastically shed pounds by cutting down calorie intake without going on any crazy diets. In fact, it is possible to keep your normal calorie intake while still following this lifestyle.

## Getting Started with Intermittent Fasting

One of the things that you need to do is to adjust your eating habits. You will not be depriving your body of food or nutrition. Instead, you will be eating much later or earlier than usual. This lifestyle simply requires you to deny yourself food and nourishment for a couple of hours during the day or night.

While this process can seem daunting at first, what you need to do is to approach it using the following steps.

- o Breakdown the fasting process into small yet simple, doable steps
- o Simple step-by-step actions will guarantee success
- o Make observations at each stage then analyze the observation
- o Come up with a conclusion about the observation and analysis

However, before you get started, there are a couple of things that you need to. You should first speak with a healthcare expert such as a doctor.

**1. Speak to a doctor before starting:** It is absolutely important to speak to your physician about this lifestyle before you begin. Your doctor will assess your health and advice about any medical condition you may have. Generally, if you are pregnant, are lactating, have a chronic condition or other issues of concern, then your doctor will advise you appropriately.

**2. Keep it simple:** It is advisable to keep things as simple as possible. When you fast, you are allowed to take water, black coffee, unsweetened tea, or green tea.

**3. Take it easy:** Try and eat your normal meals when you are not fasting. For best outcomes, try and focus on low carb diets, whole foods, fruits, and vegetables. Also, remember to stay hydrated. At this juncture, you will want to launch a program that has great chances of success. Your goal really should be to get to the end of your fast successfully.

**4. Time:** Do not be too blinded by days or time. These are provided only as a guide. For instance, you do not have to start or complete your fasts at a fixed time, say 10.00 am or 2.00 pm. You can choose to follow indicated times but generally, you should set times and choose days that best suit you and your lifestyle.

**5. Best day of the week:** It is up to you to choose which days of the week that you will fast. Fasting on weekdays is more convenient compared to weekends because these are structured. Most people prefer to fast on Mondays, Wednesdays, or Thursdays. Try not to fast on consecutive days.

**6. Slip-ups are fine:** Sometimes we fail in our quests to follow this lifestyle. If you forget to fast or consume too many calories, do not despair. Some people are prone to giving in. basically, just do what you need to do and then get back on track.

# Additional steps to get you started

## 1. Determine what your fasting goal is

You need to first determine what your fasting goals are. What is the purpose you wish to achieve through intermittent fasting? For some, it could be weight loss and weight maintenance. Fasting has been proven to reduce some hormones such as insulin while increasing others like HGH or the human growth hormone and norepinephrine.

You can decide to fast in order to relieve symptoms of a certain illness or even to avoid medication. Fasting can help you to better manage chronic conditions such as heart disease and diabetes and even internal inflammation. It is great for preventing serious diseases while increasing longevity.

## 2. Address all your fears and worries

It is common to have concerns, questions, and worries, especially when embarking on a journey. It is also possible that there are aspects of intermittent fasting that bother you. If so, then you should address all these fears, as answers are available to them all.

**Can I skip breakfast?** Absolutely, you really don't have to have breakfast and it is not the most important meal of the day. Numerous dieters view it as a neutral meal which won't affect your life much. For instance, it will not cause you to lose weight nor will it fire up your metabolism.

**Should I avoid snacks?** If you wish to skip snacks then that is okay. Snacking is generally allowed as part of intermittent fasting but not snacking is also okay. It is a habit that won't cause you to lose weight, as it does not boost metabolism. However, unplanned snacking can contribute to liver disease and obesity. Metabolism will not slow down. It is a known fact that fasting does increase your metabolism. When your metabolism rate increases, then you will increase and retain your muscle mass even as you lose weight.

## Other Crucial Considerations

- ○ *Choose your preferred fasting protocol*

There are a number of different fasting protocols out there. Study them closely and see which ones are the most suitable for your lifestyle. It will be much easier for you if you get a protocol that is in tune with your lifestyle.

For example, if you are more of a morning person who enjoys working hard in the morning and enjoying a snack thereafter, then identify the protocol that is close to this lifestyle. Others love to work out in the evening so find which one will generally match your lifestyle.

If you choose to fast two days a week, then choose days such as Mondays and Wednesdays or Tuesdays and Thursdays. This way, you will be able to fast with little distraction compared to fasting over the weekend when there are parties, visits, family members and so on.

You can choose the eat-stop-eat protocol in this instance. This means that on your fasting days, you will fast for 16 hours each day and then have all your meals and snacks within the 8-hour eating window. You will mostly consume not more than 500 calories for women and 600 calories for men on your fasting days. On other days, you will aim for 2200 – 2400 for women and 2400 – 2600 for men on your other days.

There are a couple of other factors that you will need to consider when choosing your preferred protocol. For instance, are you trying to lose weight, fast for the long term, or for religious reasons? If you can answer these questions, then you will be able to clearly choose the most appropriate protocol that is aligned with your lifestyle. You will be more flexible if your reasons for fasting include anti-aging, building lean muscle or longevity and so on.

o **Adjust your eating habits**

You should start considering adjusting your eating habits at this stage. The attractive aspect of intermittent fasting is the fact that it does not dictate what foods to eat but rather when to eat and when to fast.

However, you should choose healthy, natural foods rather than junk food or highly processed foods. A healthy diet and occasional workouts are necessary for weight loss and a healthy body. Unhealthy foods such as junk food will leave you feeling lethargic and will not support your weight loss ambitions.

o **Conduct sufficient research all the time**

Intermittent fasting has numerous health benefits. However, it has a number of protocols. You need to identify one of these protocols and then make a determination about it. You should really be guided by your lifestyle when choosing a particular protocol to follow.

## Now Begin the Transition

Now that you have a lot of relevant information, you should begin intermittent fasting. Ensure that you ease gently into your preferred protocol. You may find that it involves delaying your first of the day as much as possible. You should avoid late night eating or snacking.

## Hydration is Crucial as You Fast

You need to stay hydrated as you fast. Water is crucial for the body and a major necessity for numerous processes. You need to stay hydrated so that normal processes proceed without a hitch.

Water hydrates the body. It also plays other crucial roles. For instance, it is used to eliminate toxins from the body and this is why some experts believe that you should drink plenty of water even as you fast. Some say that you should drink at least 8 glasses each day.

On top of frequent water drinking, you need to take plenty of other beverages. These include unsweetened tea, green tea, and black coffee. These beverages help to keep you hydrated as well as fight off hunger pangs.

Remember to spread your hydration throughout the day. If you drink too much water all at once, you will not hydrate properly as you will eliminate most of it almost immediately.

## How to Overcome Hunger Pangs

If you wish to overcome hunger pangs as you fast, then you need to make deliberate stops to avoid feeling hungry. Hunger can be both physiological and physical. If you manage to conquer hunger especially in the early days, then you will be alright.

**1. Ensure that you have the right mindset:** you need to understand and appreciate that fasting is real and that you are likely to feel hungry especially at the onset. You need to keep in mind that you are not likely to suffer any setbacks because of fasting. If you start feeling hungry just at the onset of fasting, then you should not give in and think that it is not possible. Instead, you should hold out for as long as you can. Also, you should not be fantasizing about your next meal or snack. Instead, you should keep busy and focus on your work and other things. You should also think about all the benefits you stand to gain by fasting regularly.

**2. Understand that there is real hunger and psychological hunger.** There are two distinct types of hunger. There is the general hunger that we feel after abstaining from food for a long period of time. Physical hunger can be satiated with food. However, you may also suffer from psychological hunger. Emotional or psychological hunger is different. It results from many causes such as stress, emotional pain, guilt, worry, and so on. Psychological hunger keeps you craving for more and more food especially the processed kind. You usually feel uncomfortably full after eating and this makes you feel guilty.

**3. Keep both your mind and body active:** Being active is crucial as it keeps your mind focused elsewhere. If you are not busy then you will focus on the hunger pains and keep thinking about food. Therefore, try and focus on things other than food. For instance, if you are employed, then try and focus on the work at hand. You should immerse yourself in activities even when you are not working. When you are generally busy and with constant flow, then you will notice that time flies very fast. Being busy also helps you to lose weight.

**4. Take a tablespoon or two of Psyllium Husk:** Psyllium Husk is an edible type of soluble fiber and has numerous benefits for the body. It also serves as a prebiotic which is excellent for the digestive system. This is why it is often used as a dietary supplement. When you take this product regularly or as advised, it will draw water from your colon and sweep it clean of all waste. You will stop feeling full or bloated. Psyllium is known to promote a healthy heart and it has a positive effect on cholesterol levels.

**5. Battling hunger as you fast:** As you progress along your intermittent fasting journey, you will note that hunger is only a problem during the initial stages. As soon as your body begins to get used to the change, it will be easier for you to cope. You should expect to suffer serious hunger pangs for the first two to three weeks. After the fourth week, hunger will cease to be a major issue.

# Things You Need to Unlearn

Research conducted by various institutions has opened our eyes to certain truths. There is a lot of misinformation out there. A lot of people currently have the wrong misinformation about calorie intake, type of foods to eat, and so much more. Here are a couple of things that we need to unlearn.

## 1. We need to eat six small meals per day spread throughout the day

There was a time that people strongly believed in having six complete meals each day. These include breakfast, tea, lunch, a snack, dinner, and dessert. We all thought that this is how we ought to live. Fortunately, we have now learned through research that we can survive without snacks. We can also survive on 2 to 3 meals per day.

## 2. Fasting can cause you serious harm

There is a popular belief that claims fasting or nutrition deprivation can have serious health consequences even after a short while. Well, we now know differently. Fasting is common among many communities around the world. It has been practiced for centuries with excellent results. The truth is that fasting will not do you any harm but it will help you overcome many challenges you may be facing. Fasting can help you combat diseases, illnesses and also keep you looking young and healthy.

## 3. Breakfast is the most crucial meal of the day

We have for a long time been of the opinion that breakfast is essential and must be had each morning. This has now been established to be false. We do not need to have breakfast at all. It is an optional meal that we can do without. Breakfast is also not the most crucial meal of the day. You can, therefore, choose whether to have breakfast or skip it regularly.

## 4. Late night eating is bad for you

For a long time, we have been told not to eat late in the night. Many people believe that late night eating will make you fat and cause you to add weight. The reasoning is that the calories from your late-night meal or midnight snack will be stored as fat as you do not engage in any activities as you sleep. However, that is not how it works. The body does not care what time you eat. What matters is the total number of calories consumed. Therefore, do not be too concerned about when you eat but rather the total number of calories per day.

### 5. All fats are bad for you

Fats, together with carbs, have long been castigated as bad for the body. People generally believe that fats are not healthy and are bad for you. They are stored all over the body and are thought to clog the arteries. It is true that saturated fats and trans fats are bad for you. They are the ones found in packaged foods and snacks and can negatively affect your health and weight.

However, monounsaturated and polyunsaturated fats are actually really good for the body when taken in moderation. These oils are found in nuts, olives, fatty fish, and avocados. They are good for your heart and brain and great for the skin. They are absolutely essential for any healthy diet and are great for your health too. It is therefore quite okay to enjoy a healthy dose of fatty foods every day just as long as these are monounsaturated and polyunsaturated fats.

## Intermittent Fasting and Exercise

If you truly want to reap the maximum benefits from the fasting lifestyle, then you should ensure that you engage in regular exercises and workouts. For effective exercises, you should consider coming up with a work out regime. However, things can get tricky when you are fasting because of energy levels. You will need to take some precautions if you are to exercise in a fasted state. Here are a couple of things that you can consider.

## 1. Plan your meals around your workouts

If you want to lose a lot of weight very fast, then you may want to do is workout on an empty stomach. What this means is that you will work out before having anything to eat. This can be tricky at first so you should plan your meals accordingly. However, it is a very effective weight loss plan.

You can wake up in the morning and probably go for a jog, a swim, or do some cardio workouts. However, you should ensure that you eat the right kind of foods the night before. For instance, you should have some complex carbs and protein. These will help you build your glycogen stores with the right kind of energy. If you do this you will have sufficient energy for your workouts.

Try never to work out on a full stomach. All you need to ensure that you do is to plan early, think about your workouts and what time you wish to work out. The crucial point that you need to note is that your nutrition needs should match the demands of your workouts even when you have to work out early in the morning.

## 2. Use the best approach

Basically, whenever you work out, you should do so to your heart's content. However, you should stop if you start feeling dizzy, lightheadedness or sick. This can occur whenever you are fasting. Things will get easier once you get used to fasting. Try and start out with less taxing workouts and light exercises especially if you are not used to fasting. If you do so, then your blood sugar levels will drop to serious levels and you may start feeling dizzy.

Remember to pay attention to your body and listen to what it says. If you feel sick or weak, stop and take a break. You can always work out at a different time. Also, a little planning goes a long so always remember to plan ahead and prepare adequately before your workouts.

## Things that You are Allowed to Have

### 1. Black Coffee

You are allowed to drink Black coffee as you fast. Having this in your fasted state helps to reduce appetite and stave off hunger. Coffee also accelerates metabolism and has a positive effect on your strength and stamina.
If you don't like Black coffee and alternative can be Zero sugar energy drinks that have no calories. This is not recommended however if you need a kick of energy during your fast, this is an alternative.

### 2. Water

You should take plenty of water. Water is essential as it performs important functions in the body. It is funny though because most people forget to drink sufficient amounts of water yet this is a simple requirement. people avoid drinking water because it has a flat taste and keeps sending them to the bathroom. However, water flushes toxins from your body and leaves you well hydrated. It also keeps you feeling full and you do not have to worry about feeling hungry.

### 3. Green tea

If you do not like the taste of water, then you can add a slice of lemon to improve the taste. Lemon does not just improve the taste of water but also helps to kill off germs in your system. Alternatively, you can opt for green tea.

Apparently, green tea is excellent for you even as you fast. Green tea dramatically reduces hunger pangs and enables you to stay focused on the task ahead rather than your next meal. Green tea contains catechins which are effective in burning fat, especially stubborn tummy fat.

Green tea also contains powerful antioxidants that help with detoxification. It supports autophagy which is the body's own cleansing mechanism. Green tea also helps to eliminate free radicals which are very harmful to the body. Therefore, always have a cup of green tea handy as you fast.

*Bone broth?* There are suggestions that bone broth is ideal when you are fasting. Bone broth contains very few calories but is excellent in your fasted state. It contains some micronutrients that provide you with energy. If you get to feel very hungry, then you should warm a cup and have it in your fasted state.

# Chapter 4: Counting Your Calorie Intake

## What are Macronutrients?

Macronutrients can be defined as nutrients that provide the body with energy or calories. Nutrients are chemicals or substances that are essential for certain functions in the body such as metabolism and growth.

Macronutrients are needed in large amounts and this is why we use the term "macro". Macro means large or huge. There are three major macronutrients that are essential to humans. These are;

- Lipids
- Proteins
- Carbohydrates

There are certain quantities of calories that we receive when we eat foods from each group. Carbohydrates and proteins provide 4 calories per gram while fat provides 9 calories per gram. Alcohol provides 7 calories per gram. However, it is not a macronutrient and is not essential for life.

Humans need macronutrients, water, and micronutrients for survival. Micronutrients are essential nutrients that our bodies required in smaller amounts. They include minerals and vitamins.

***Proteins:*** We need to consume proteins each and every day. According to health recommendations, we need to ensure that between 10% and 35% of all the calories that we consume. All human cells contain protein and it constitutes a major part of our organs, muscles, glands, muscles, and the skin.

***Carbohydrates:*** according to science, our bodies need carbohydrates in the largest amount compared to other macronutrients. Of all the calories we consume daily, about 45% to 65% should be from carbohydrates. There are a number of reasons why carbohydrates are so crucial. Here are those reasons.

- o        Carbohydrates are the body's most crucial source of energy
- o        They are easily absorbed by the body
- o        Are crucial for waste elimination and intestinal health
- o        Are easily stored in the liver and muscles for future energy use
- o        Are essential in muscles, brain, kidneys, nervous system, heart

Almost all living organisms, both animals and plants, do contain some carbohydrates. Even then, it is easier to obtain them from some sources compared to others. For instance, starches are a great source of carbohydrates. Examples of starches are;

- o     Cereal grains such as rice, barley, wheat, millet, and oats
     Fruits like bananas, grapes, plums, cherries, dates, apricots,   melons, apples, etc.
- o     Legumes such as peas, lentils, beans, and peanuts
     Starchy vegetables such as pumpkin, yams, cassava root,        potatoes, etc.
- o     Mildly starchy veggies such as cauliflower, beets, carrots, salsify

***Fats:*** A lot of people have negative thoughts about fats and fatty oils. This is because they are blamed for weight gain. However, fats are essential for human survival. The recommended daily fat intake is 20% to 33% of all the calories that you consume.

Fat consists of individual fatty acids. These fatty acids are generally the building blocks that fats are made of. Some of the most useful fatty acids in the body are omega-3 and omega-6. These are also known as essential fatty acids. They are important mainly for two reasons mostly. They are used in the production of substances that control chemical reactions in the cells and also help in the formation of cell membranes or outer layer of cells. Fats are essential for the following purposes;

- They provide organs with cushioning
- Are essential for normal growth and development
- Fats are needed for absorption of fat-soluble vitamins
- Are an excellent source of energy
- They make food stable, consistent, and tasty
- They help to maintain cell membranes

**Fiber:** This is a carbohydrate that is not digested by the body. This carbohydrate passes through the alimentary canal and aids in waste elimination. It is advisable to consume foods that are high in fiber as they have been shown to reduce the risks of obesity and high disease. They have also been proven to lower high cholesterol. Such foods include whole grains, vegetables, and fruits.

*Putting this information to use*

- Bake or grill your food rather than fry it
- Choose smoked mackerel instead of some greasy fry-up
- Always choose lean meat such as fish and chicken over steaks
- Choose sauces made out of tomatoes
- Grate cheese if you have to so as to make it last longer

When you work so hard and watch what you eat in order to lose weight, you probably assume others have the same knowledge. If

45

you don't then you could possibly be fumbling in the dark. Some of the most crucial steps you will need to follow include working out more and learning how to count calories and use a food tracker.

***Calories do not represent nutrition but energy***
When you fill your plate with food, it is only the calories do not give a full picture of what's going on but just part of it. Calories are an indicator of the amount of energy that you eat. However, they do not paint a full picture of the quality or nutrition that you take.

When you count calories, you are able to receive the correct amount of energy that your body needs and also ensure that you work towards your weight loss goals.

# Counting Macronutrients

All the food that we eat consists of three macros. These are protein, carbohydrates, and fats. They are the building blocks of the food we eat. There is a difference, however, between tracking macros and counting calories. If you only count macros then you could lose out on crucial nutrients.

## Tracking macros
Tracking macros encourage a healthier choice of food types. When you track your macros, you will be able to determine the quality of your calories. You will ensure that your foods come from all the three major sources of calories. Tracking macros are good for you. There are rations available that have been determined by nutrition bodies such as the Food and Nutrition Board of the IOM or institution of Medicine.

If you want to eat healthy as per the recommendations of the Food and Nutrition Board, then you should aim to have 20 – 35% of your diet in the form of fats, 10 – 35% proteins, and 45% -

65% carbs. I recommend going low carbs and high fats and proteins if you want to lose more fat and build more muscle.

## How to Track Macronutrients

It is crucial that you learn how to track the macronutrients – proteins, carbohydrates, and fats. By tracking these important nutrients, you will be able to consume a well-balanced diet on a regular basis and also attain your specific dietary goals.

Counting macronutrients, especially for homemade meals is pretty simple. You will need to follow a step-by-step procedure in order to attain your goals. All you need to do to successfully work out your macronutrient intake is to answer two questions. You will need to be able to break down your food to the macronutrient level and then determine how much of it you want to eat.

### 1. Identify the different food items in your meal

If your meal comes packaged with a label, then you can skip this step. However, if you prepared the meal from scratch at home, then you will need to make a note of each item in the meal. Get a piece of paper or even a tabulated sheet such as an Excel or Google sheet. Your meal could, for instance, include zucchini, onions, tomatoes, garlic, and some extra virgin olive oil. List all these food items down.

### 2. Calculate the quantity of each food serving for those with labels

If you purchase pre-packed food, then you should be able to see the serving sizes. Simply take the quantity that you consumed and divide this by the serving size. Once you get the answer, you will then determine the individual macronutrients in the food in order to determine how much of each you ate.

### 3. Make use of the USDA Food Search tool

Use the chart described to determine the levels of calories in your food. Fresh fruits and vegetables are often referred to as "raw foods" as they are unprocessed. You can also use the search tool to determine the quantity that best represents the amount of each macronutrient on your plate.

Once you are able to break down your food into macros and then determine the amount of each on your plate, you will be able to work out the calorie content of each. Using the Food Search tool is pretty easy if you have the right information.

Now sum up all the protein in your plate, all the carbohydrates, and all the fats. You will find figures or values such as total protein = 48.6 grams, total carbohydrates = 238.4 grams and total fats = 62.6 grams. Now you need to convert these figures into calories. This is pretty simple because we already know the amount of calories in each macronutrient.

### Use a food tracker application program or App

Alternatively, you can use a food tracker app. If you find that tracking macronutrients are a little challenging, then you can use an application program or app. Rather than calculating your TDEE or total daily energy expenditure, you can use a health tracker to work this out for you.

Using a food tracker helps to save you time, eliminates any guesswork, and provides you with more detailed figures than you need. Some of these apps have macro-based meal plans so that you do not have to be concerned about how to increase carbohydrate levels while keeping other macronutrients the same.

## Calculating Macros for Weight Loss
In order to work out the necessary macros for weight loss, you need to determine your TDEE or total daily energy expenditure. This is simply the total amount of calories or energy that you

expend each day. If you want to lose weight, you will eat less and less food each day.

There is a basic formula used to calculate your TDEE. In fact, there are plenty of formulae. However, the most important one used today is known as the Mifflin St. Jeor formula.

Resting energy expenditure (REE): This is the energy that your body uses when you are resting.

Males: REE = 10 X weight (kg) + 6.25 X height (cm) − 5X age(yrs) + 5

Females: REE = 10 X weight (kg) + 6.25 X height (cm) − 5X age (yrs) − 161

However, most people do not just sit down all day. They engage in one activity or the other. Therefore, once you work out the REE, you can then determine the TDEE of individuals based on their physical activity.

Sedentary lifestyle: TDEE = REE X 1.2
Light activity:       TDEE = REE X 1.375
Moderate activity:    TDEE = REE X 1.55
Very active:          TDEE = REE X 1.725

### *An example of how to work out your calories*
Let us assume that you are a 30-year-old man weighing 80kg, 184 cm, who is moderately active. This is the equation that will determine how much calories you consume each day.

[10 X weight (kg) + 6.25 x height (cm)] − [5 X age (yrs) + 5 = REE] X 1.55

(10 X 80) + (6.25 X 184) − (5 X 30) + 5 = REE
800 + 1150 − 150 + 5 = 1805

Since you are moderately active, we will multiply the REE X 1.55 = 2797 calories

Therefore, based on your activity level and body measurements, you will consume about 2797 calories per day. For weight loss purposes, you should shed your calories by not more than 20%. For weight maintenance, eat calories equivalent to your TDEE. However, if you eat more calories than this, then you will definitely gain weight.

### *Tracking your Macros*

If you wish to track your calories, then experts advise that you use a suitable app or application program. There are plenty of reliable ones out there. One that comes highly recommended is known as MyFitnessApp. It is available on both Android and iOS platforms. You can also use the MyMacros+ which is even more flexible and has a lot more variables and options for you.

Alternatively, you can buy and use a food scale. While plenty of nutritional information is available on food packaging, you can still use a food scale which is a lot more accurate. Using a food scale will ensure that you are accurately tracking the food that you eat.

# Best Time to Work Out when Fasting

There are no specific work out times because people have different preferences. However, it has been shown that working out early in the morning on an empty stomach is the best for weight loss. Even health experts recommend working out on an empty stomach.

You can go for an early morning jog or gym work out. If you plan to work out in the morning, and then ensure that you eat a suitable dinner the night before. Complex carbohydrates should be part of your dinner because they release energy slowly.

Then we have fasted workouts or fasted cardio. This is when you work out during your fasting period. It is one of the best approaches for anyone looking to lose weight. However, you need to be careful whenever you opt for fasted cardio. Your body can be depleted of energy reserves and this will leave you feeling weak and dizzy. It is advisable to avoid fasted workouts until your body gets used to the fasting lifestyle.

# Chapter 5: Health Benefits of Intermittent Fasting

There are numerous health benefits of intermittent fasting. These include physical benefits, mental, and physiological. It is a fact that what is good for the body is also good for your brain as well. While on the major benefits of intermittent fasting is weight loss, there are plenty of other benefits throughout the body.

Intermittent fasting not only helps with weight loss but also helps to improve certain metabolic features that are great for the brain. These include lower insulin resistance and reduced blood sugar levels, reduced inflammation and lower levels of oxidative stress.

To understand the benefits of intermittent fasting, it is important to also appreciate what happens to the body when we fast especially at cellular level. When you fast, your body does not have all the food it needs to produce energy. However, the body must have energy. Therefore, the liver begins breaking down amino acids and fats into glucose. Your energy levels will reduce as the body begins conserving energy.

A process known as ketosis will begin. At this stage, the body will begin to burn stored fats to produce energy. As soon as it sets in, you will then stop feeling hungry or lightheadedness. At the same time, your blood pressure will fall and the heart rate will slow down. Ketosis is excellent for balancing blood sugar and promoting weight loss and other physiological benefits.

# Evidence-Based Benefits of Intermittent Fasting

### 1. You lose weight and stubborn belly fat

One of the major benefits of intermittent fasting is that you lose weight and shed off the pounds. This is because the body will stop relying on food to produce energy as you fast and instead reach into fat reserves. Therefore, when you start fasting, you begin a slow but steady weight loss process. As you keep this lifestyle up, you will notice further weight loss. Expect to lose anywhere between 3% and 8% of your total body weight in just 3 to 24 weeks.

### 2. It supports the regulation of functions of genes, hormones, and cells

There is clear research-based evidence showing that intermittent fasting regulates hormones in the body and also ensures superior hormonal balance. As you fast, the organs get to rest and this includes the liver which is a crucial organ necessary for balancing hormones.

**Insulin:** this is a hormone that is released by the pancreas. Its function is to regulate the sugar levels in the blood. As you fast, the body starts converting stored fats into energy in order to fuel cell activity. As the body loses more fat, it becomes more responsive to insulin and it gets absorbed more.

Better absorption of insulin in the body results in better blood sugar regulation. This helps to prevent diabetes or manage it such that sometimes patients may not need to use medication. Thus intermittent fasting offers an excellent solution that helps prevent diabetes. Insulin resistance is a situation that occurs due to excessive glucose in the blood.

**Human growth hormone:** HGH or human growth hormone is responsible for multiplication and division of cells. It also promotes and stimulates the synthesis of collagen in skeletal muscles and tendons. HGH improves your physical performance and boosts your immune system. Fasting boosts HGH levels in the blood by almost 5 times. It has numerous benefits to the body including the development of strong bones, lean muscle, healthy hair growth and so much more.

**Cortisol:** It is also known as the stress hormone. It is supplied to the body when it is stressed. This is why it is also known as the fight or flight hormone. It triggers just that kind of response. This stress hormone is properly regulated by regular fasting. When insulin is properly managed, very little cortisol is released into the body.

**Estrogen:** The female hormone estrogen can cause issues such as weight gain, irritability, and headaches if it is present in large numbers. An enzyme known as aromatase, found in most tissues, converts testosterone into estrogen. This enzyme is prevalent in fatty cells so individuals with high-fat levels usually have elevated estrogen levels. Low-fat levels in the body reduce the presence of aromatase and in return estrogen levels will reduce.

**Cells:** Cells provide storage space for fats and sometimes dangerous pathogens. During fasting sessions, your body reaches out the cells and utilizes the stored fat. In the process, the body also consumes or eliminates all pathogens found in such cells. Also, the cells get renewed and rejuvenated with newer cells produced that are more efficient, fat-free, effective, and efficient.

### 3. Intermittent fasting enhances metabolism
When you fast, you provide the digestive system with relief. Regular fasting tends to boost metabolism which ensures that the body burns fat more efficiently. Fasting combined with regular exercises provide the best way of losing weight, shedding fat and keeping it off, becoming fit and so on. Intermittent fasting enhances metabolism by cleansing the cells on the inside. It also helps to regulate your digestive system and metabolic action. In the process, it also promotes healthy bowel function and also improves the metabolic action.

The minute that your metabolism slows down, the aging process will begin. This is why an efficient metabolism keeps aging at bay. Fasting provides your digestive system a break from the usual grind of digestion. Again, when you improve your eating habits by eating the right foods in the right quantity, you will energize your metabolism so that it becomes efficient and functions as required.

### 4. It reduces the risk of type II diabetes

One of the most serious chronic conditions is type II diabetes. It is a condition or disease that occurs due to excessive amounts of blood sugar in the body. Our bodies usually produce insulin in order to help regulate blood sugar levels. However, levels of blood sugar can increase greatly such that the insulin levels cannot manage it. Diabetes is usually the result of excessive blood sugar levels that cannot be managed. When the body becomes resistant to insulin, then glucose will accumulate in tissues not designed for fat storage.

Intermittent fasting has been proven to reduce blood sugar levels and keep them down to manageable levels for the short, medium, and long terms. With fasting comes a drastic reduction of blood sugar levels as well as excessive fats. You can expect a reduction in blood sugar levels of between 3% and 6% once you start fasting. Therefore, fasting can have a major and positive effect on blood sugar levels.

### 5. Intermittent fasting boosts your immune system

One of the crucial systems in the body is the immune system. It provides you with protection against dangerous pathogens, diseases, and infections of all kinds. According to research by scientists at the University of Southern California, fasting can help to regenerate the immune system. It achieves this by triggering the production of new white cells that fight off infections keeping you free from infections and diseases.

Fasting allows your body to eliminate inefficient, worn out, and damaged cells that constitute your immunity system. Researchers believe that intermittent fasting can assist anyone with low immunity to boost their levels in order to prevent infections and stay healthy.

## 6. Intermittent fasting helps to extend lifespan
There is a strong correlation between intermittent fasting and longevity. Researchers at the University of Chicago in Illinois have discovered that intermittent fasting can delay the development of disorders that usually lead to death. The research has shown that individuals who practice regular fasting do benefit from healthier and longer life compared to those who don't. When your digestive system and metabolic activity are constantly working, then you set in motion the aging process. Fasting produces the opposite reaction. It results in stress within the cells which promotes cell and tissue repair. These anti-aging properties assist in keeping your organs functioning effectively and efficiently.

## 7. It is excellent for brain health
Your brain is an extremely important organ of the body. Scientists say that what is good for the body is good for the brain. As you fast, your metabolism rates will improve greatly. Improved metabolism helps to reduce oxidative stress, inflammation, and blood sugar levels. According to a report released in 2015 by the Society for Neuroscientists, the brain gets stimulated in different ways. The study shows that intermittent fasting has major benefits for the brain.

When the brain is stimulated, your memory will be enhanced in various ways. Also, this will enhance recovery after an injury while promoting the growth of neurons. Fasting promotes conditions of the brain so that risks of brain conditions such as Parkinson's and Alzheimer's. The research scientists behind this study also claim the fasting improves quality of life as well as cognitive functions of patients with these brain problems.

## 8. It helps to combat oxidative stress
Oxidative stress is a type of stress that is usually caused by unstable molecules in the body. These unstable molecules are also known as free radicals. These can be extremely dangerous to

56

the body. They cause serious damage to organs and enhance the aging process. They are also thought to play a huge role in the development and onset of cancer and other health conditions.

Intermittent fasting provides an excellent solution to these problems and challenges. Research findings show that regular fasting provides a solution to the challenges posed by free radicals. Basically, as you fast, you activate your stress defenses. These defenses are activated in the body even in the absence of the stressor. As the body begins to break down fats as you fast, it begins to eliminate waste and toxins present in your body. Once cells are cleaned, the rejuvenation process of these cells begins. Fasting will also promote or help to battle inflammation.

### 9. Intermittent fasting is beneficial to your heart
According to statistics, heart disease is the world's top killer. Millions of Americans will expect to fall victims to heart disease. Some of the risk factors associated with a healthy heart include blood pressure, LDL cholesterol, and others.

Research scientists are of the opinion that regular checkups are essential and it also helps you lose weight. Fasting helps to eliminate bad cholesterol. All these are factors that need to be considered as high-risk indicators of heart disease. When you fast and work out regularly, then these will help lower your risk levels. Reduced bodyweight helps you to be flexible and move fast.

With lower body fat and weight, you are able to move faster and the risk of heart disease will be greatly reduced. It is widely believed that any person who pursues this kind of lifestyle like you and others do will have a healthier heart.

Doctors have known for a long time that individuals who follow a restricted calorie intake once or twice a week will most certainly have better heart health compared to those who do not.

# Health Benefits of Calorie Restrictions

There are numerous credible studies that confirm the benefits of calorie restrictions on human health. According to the findings of some of these studies, not only do you benefit from calorie restrictions but that this is an essential requirement if you are to live a long healthy life.

Research done on mice at the John Hopkins University clearly indicates that life-long calorie restriction significantly alters the general structure of gut bacteria or microbiota. This alteration happens in a manner that tends to promote longevity. Therefore, calorie restriction promotes longevity by altering the structure of gut microbiota.

Longevity due to calorie restrictions is more a factor of a reduction in disease states within the body that would otherwise destroy life. There are certain health improvements that are also associated with calorie restrictions. They include improved insulin sensitivity, lower visceral fat levels, lower blood pressure, and reduced inflammation levels.

Intermittent fasting shares similar benefits to calorie restrictions even when you do not strictly restrict daily calorie intake. A review was conducted by research scientists in 2013 at the University of Chicago. This review revealed a wide range of therapeutic benefits that were as a result of intermittent fasting. These benefits are actually possible even when there was no significant reduction in the total amount of calories consumed. In reality, if you choose a specific intermittent fasting protocol, you will still be able to consume the same amount of calories each day like before and still enjoy the benefits of intermittent fasting.

**Intermittent Fasting Helps with the Following**

- It reduces inflammation
- Lowers blood pressure
- Reduces levels of dangerous visceral fats

- Causes stem cells to start the self-renewal process
- Protects the body against cardiovascular diseases
- Improves the functions of the pancreas
- Activates reduction in oxidative stress and cellular damage
- Prevents or slows down the progression of type II diabetes
- Significantly reduces body weight for overweight and obese persons
- Improves your metabolic efficiency

## Advice and Tips for Successful Intermittent Fasting

Drink green tea during fasting. While not essential, it makes the experience easier. Green tea suppresses appetite and curbs hunger pangs.

It is important to drink water when you fast as it will fill your stomach. This sends a message to the brain that you are full and you will feel less hungry.

Be on the lookout for body cues. For instance, if you feel upset or stressed out during your fast, then try and relax. Take some deep breaths and focus closely because this is exactly what hunger does to you.

Stock your house with plenty of healthy foods and snacks. These can include grains, veggies, and lean proteins. If you do this, then you will always feed your body the healthy stuff instead of binging on the wrong food types.

# Chapter 6: Food Guide

Intermittent Fasting is a lifestyle that involves a pattern of fasting and eating. It is, therefore, more than just a diet. This lifestyle does not dictate what you should eat but rather when you should have your meals. Even then, if you wish to benefit from this lifestyle, then you really should focus on what you eat.

Changing what you eat is crucial because you will be able to lose weight and gain lean muscle without necessarily having to drastically cut back on your calorie intake. Some dieters prefer having large meals within a shorter period of time. This is, in fact, an excellent way of losing weight while maintaining your muscle mass.

## Food and Nutrition

Nutrition is simply the science about the nutrients found in foods and the relationship between these nutrients and growth, reproduction, good health, and disease.

According to Lauren Harris-Pincus, MS, RDN, who is also the author of "The Protein-Packed Breakfast Club", if you want to enjoy all the benefits of intermittent fasting then you should resort to clean eating. This means eating fresh foods, natural produce, whole grains, and lean meats as often as possible.

### Nutrient-Dense Foods
Experts agree that having a well-balanced diet is essential for weight loss and maintaining energy levels. It is also crucial if you are to stick with this lifestyle. Therefore, if you want to be healthy, lose weight, and enjoy all other benefits of intermittent fasting, then you should focus on eating nutrient-dense foods.

These include seeds, beans, nuts, veggies, fruits, whole grains as well as lean proteins and dairy products.

Your target really should be foods that improve health such as unprocessed foods, those rich in fiber, whole foods, and foods that offer flavor and variety. Therefore, ensure that you eat from a wide range of foods. Here is a list of some of these foods.

**Water:** While you may not be eating for most of the day, you should still hydrate your body. All the organs in your body really need water in order to function optimally. While the amount of water than people drink varies, you should aim at having urine that is a pale yellow color at all times. Should the color be dark yellow then it means that you are dehydrated.

If you do get dehydrated, then you are likely to suffer from fatigue, headaches, and dizziness. This is even worse when you are fasting so always ensure that you stay hydrated at all times. Should you not like the taste of water, then you can add a slice of lemon or cucumber or perhaps a few mint leaves.

**Cruciferous vegetables:** One of the crucial ingredients for your diet is fiber. This is found in plenty in cruciferous vegetables like cauliflower, Brussels sprouts, and broccoli. Fiber is essential for eliminating waste, preventing constipation, and keeping your digestive system in excellent working condition. Fiber also makes you feel full so you do not need to snack throughout the day.

**Fish:** You should aim to eat at least 8 ounces of fish each week or more if possible. There are great reasons why this is important. Fish is not just delicious but is excellent for your health. This is because it contains a number of excellent nutrients such as vitamin D, vitamin E, proteins, and other healthy oils like omega-3 fatty acids. If you will be fasting most of the day, then you will be better off with a food that provides maximum nutrition. Fish is also considered a "brain food" as it provides the brain with essential nutrients required for optimum performance.

**Avocado:** One reason that avocados are so popular is because they contain plenty of good fats. While some may wonder why choose a fruit with so many calories when weight loss is the goal, this is a very satiating food. Also, the oils contained in avocado fruit are monounsaturated. This means that they are great for the body. Avocado will keep you feeling full most of the day so you can go about your business even if you are fasting.

**Berries:** If you love smoothies, then you probably top them up with fruit. One of the most nutritious yet delicious fruits out there is the berry. You have a wide range of berries to choose from. They range from strawberries to blueberries and all others. They all happen to be a great source of vitamin C. Just one cup delivers more than your daily recommended allowance. There is also a recent study that found that individuals who consumed a diet rich in bio-flavanoids have very little chance of gaining weight in the immediate and long-term future. Both strawberries and blueberries are rich in bio-flavanoids among other nutrients.

**Legumes and beans:** Some of the foods best for the provision of energy include beans and legumes. While you should go slow on carbs, it doesn't hurt to have some low-calorie carbs on your menu. Think about foods such as lentils, peas, black beans, and chickpeas. Beans and legumes are definitely low-carb foods that you should have regularly. These are all known to aid with weight loss even when you simply eat normally with no calorie restrictions.

**Potatoes:** People tend to believe that all white foods are bad for you. However, some white foods such as potatoes are really great for you. Studies have shown that potatoes are very satiating. Other studies point to the fact that potatoes can actually aid with weight loss. However, if you are to benefit from potatoes then they should constitute a part of a healthy diet. You can eat them boiled, grilled, and as part of a stew. Try and avoid potato chips and French fries versions as these do not support weight loss and are not good for you.

**Whole grains:** People still find it hard to believe that you can lead a healthy lifestyle and still eat carbs. The two seem to be from totally different worlds. However, whole grains are actually excellent for your body. They are packed full of proteins and fiber. Therefore, eating just a small amount of whole grains will go a long way in getting you to feel satiated.

Studies also indicate that your metabolism is spiked up when you choose to eat whole grains instead of refined grains. You should, therefore, include whole grains as part of your regular diet. Make sure you get out of your comfort zone and try out all sorts of grains include Kamut, millet, bulgur, faro, sorghum, amaranth, spelt, and so much of what is out there. You will be surprised that whole grains actually boost your metabolism.

**Nuts:** Nuts are pretty high in calories compared to numerous other snacks. However, they contain oils that are great for the body. Good fat is what they contain and this is the difference between nuts and other snacks, most of which contain dangerous fats. In fact, research does suggest that the polyunsaturated fats in walnuts can change completely change certain markers in the body to make you feel full instead of hungry.

You should generally not worry about putting on weight due to the healthy oils in nuts. Nuts such as walnuts have much lower calories than indicated on the label. These nuts also do not get fully digested and some parts remain intact and non-absorbed.

**Eggs:** Eggs are an excellent source of protein and very nutritious. A single large contains about 6 grams of protein and can be prepared in a matter of minutes. You need to stay satiated and build muscle during the day. There is a study (https://www.ncbi.nlm.nih.gov/pubmed/20226994) which found that men who consumed an egg for breakfast rather than junk food ate less throughout the day and also felt less hungry in comparison. Therefore, next time you want to eat some awesome and filling proteins, try and remember to boil an egg.

## Include Probiotics in Your Diet

Probiotics are essential and should be included as part of your diet. They enhance the performance of the gut as well as the rest of the digestive system. The tummy loves it when you provide it with diversity and consistency.

This means that whenever you are hungry, the microbiota gut bacteria are not happy. When there are problems with the digestive system, then you will suffer from constipation and other troubles. Constipation gives you sleepless nights and terrible conditions like constipation. Fortunately, there are plenty of options out there when it comes to micro-bacteria or probiotics. If you sense problems with your digestive system, you can add foods rich in probiotics such as kombucha, kefir, and kraut.

## Foods to Avoid

There are certain foods that you need to avoid completely. While intermittent fasting does not dictate what foods you should have, there are food groups or types that you should avoid.

*1. Deep fried foods:* Deep fried foods usually lose all their nutrients. The super-hot frying oils alter the nature of foods so that they are no longer of great value to the body.

*2. Simple carbs and simple sugars:* These are often digested very fast and will cause you to feel hungry very soon thereafter. They will also spike your sugar and leave you craving for more.

*3. Processed and packaged foods:* These foods are often very low in nutrients and are never fresh. They usually contain large amounts of added sugars, plenty of salt, stabilizers, coloring, and other undesirable additives. These are definitely not good for you. If you have to have processed foods, only have it sparingly once or twice each week.

# Best Foods to Eat on Intermittent Fasting

o   Ensure that you include a serving of protein with each snack or meal. Examples of suitable proteins include grass-fed beef, chicken breast, whole eggs, Greek yogurt, chickpeas, whey protein, fish, cottage cheese, nutritional yeast, tuna, and beans.

o   You should have lots of cruciferous, green, leafy vegetables. these vegetables are packed with lots of minerals, vitamins, micronutrients, flavonoids, and others. They include cabbage, broccoli, spinach, cauliflower, lettuce, and cauliflower

o   If you feel like having a sweet snack, then opt for a fruit such as an orange than artificial sweets, candy and so on

o   Make sure that your diet includes healthy fats like olive oil, coconut oil, nut butters, nuts, grass-fed butter and so on

o   Complex carbs are excellent for your diet. These include brown rice, oats, sweet potatoes, and quinoa. These are excellent foods for weight loss

o   You should drink plenty of water throughout the day. Apart from water, you can also take green tea and coffee as you fast

# Tips about Food, Meals, and Nutrition

Intermittent fasting is a lifestyle that demands you to limit your food intake. First of all, you will need to get used to eating less than 3 meals per day on fast days. Researchers at the Longevity Institute of the University of Southern California have for the last couple of years studied meal timings, calorie restrictions, and calorie intake. According to their findings, even eating three meals per day could be too much. Basically, you will be healthier if you consume fewer meals each day. Here are some other crucial points from the experts.

**Eat breakfast or dinner, but not both:** Skipping breakfast every now and then is a great idea to introduce to your life. There are those who are completely used to breakfast and can't do without it. If that is you, then have breakfast and lunch but then skip dinner.

Fill your plate with low-calorie vegetables: low-calorie vegetables are great for you. Not only are they tasty but also fill you up and also do your body plenty of good. Also, choose high protein meals if you can. These fill you up and keep you satiated for the longest time.

**Keep your carb intake to a minimum:** Carbohydrates are pretty high in calories yet they do not leave you feeling satiated. As such, you are likely to feel hungry again pretty soon. Choose complex carbs which release energy slowly rather than simple carbs. Examples of carbs include sweet potatoes, rice, pasta, Irish potatoes, breakfast cereals, and oats and so on.

**Don't shy away from fat:** It is a fact that fats are very high in calories and are known to cause obesity. However, while fats are high in calories, they also help to make you feel full. Try and include small amounts of fats with your diet especially when you fast. The focus should be to ensure that your meals are low in carbs and sugars yet high in vegetables and proteins.

## Intermittent Fasting and Alcohol

When it comes to alcohol, it is crucial that you do not touch alcohol while fasting. You should first conclude your fasting then eat and ensure that your tummy is full before touching any alcohol. Also, ensure that you drink sufficient amounts of water because alcohol can be very dehydrating. When you hydrate, you avoid dehydration, poor athletic performance, a dry mouth, headaches, and difficulty focusing.

If you have to drink alcohol, do it during your eating window. Drinking on an empty stomach will make you drink a lot faster.

Alcohol is easily absorbed in the stomach. It is absorbed directly into the bloodstream. If you have food in your tummy it will slow down the alcohol uptake. Have a balanced meal if you are going to drink alcohol. Have this meal with your beverage to avoid getting overly intoxicated.

# Chapter 7: Getting Started with Intermittent Fasting

When you start this lifestyle change, you will need to adjust your eating habits. Intermittent fasting requires you to deny yourself food for certain times during the day. You need to keep in mind that this is a lifestyle which you will now adopt and follow. Here are some tips to help you get started.

## 1. Choose your preferred intermittent fasting protocol

There are a number of different protocols out there. They are designed to suit different dieters based on their lives. For example, if you love waking up early and working out in the morning, then you can find a fasting protocol that is best aligned with you. There are those who love working out in the evening while others during mid-morning or early afternoon.

We lead such busy lives today that we hardly have time to stop and eat. If you wish, you can fast for one or two days per week and then not worry about fasting for the rest of the week. You can, as an example, opt to fast on Monday's and Thursday's and then eat normally the rest of the week.

## 2. Adjust your eating habits

Another serious consideration you will need to make is adjusting your eating habits. While this lifestyle does not dictate the kind of foods you should eat, you should learn how to adjust your diet so that you eat mostly healthy, fresh, and nutritious foods. You also need to watch your calorie intake and avoid processed foods, junk foods, and all other unhealthy options.

Unhealthy eating can lead to undesirable effects such as high blood sugar levels, unregulated hormones, low energy levels, mood swings and so on. If you choose unhealthy food options, then your body will be forced to work extra hard in order to eliminate toxins.

### 3. Begin the Transition

You should now begin the transition. This is the transition into a lifestyle of fasting on a regular basis. Since you already have a preferred protocol, you should now begin to ease into this protocol. Easing into this protocol could be as simple as delaying your first meal of the day by a few hours and cutting back on late night eating.

You should keep in mind that intermittent fasting is a lot more about the mind than it is about diet and lifestyle. It is crucial at this stage that you adjust your chosen lifestyle. It is similar to the way muscles are trained by starting off with light weights and fewer repetitions. The weights and repetitions are then increased gradually.

Once you begin, proceed slowly but surely. The start process will involve regular adjustments of your diet, eating habits, and fasting hours. Keep improving until you get to a level that you are comfortable with.

### 4. Find a support group or person

Once you begin the intermittent fasting journey, consider finding people who share your ideals and chosen lifestyle. If you wish to be successful, then you should think about partnering with others who are on a similar lifestyle. There are plenty of places to find such support groups. Think about popular social networking sites like Facebook and Twitter.

### 5. Consider use of delayed gratification

One approach that works superbly is the delayed gratification process. Think about a child who asks the mother for permission to go out and play with other kids. Instead of a direct yes, the mother may delay approval until a later time. Basically, the delay can be used as a tool to help manage hunger and intermittent fasting. Delay eases the pain of desire.

# Reorganize your meals

It is advisable to reorganize your meals so that you eat mostly complex carbohydrates and proteins first. Some of the foods that you need to include in your diet should be fish, lean meats, fruits, vegetables, grains, and others.

You should ensure that you plan your meals on time. When you think about what you will eat later, focus on quality foods such as lean protein, white meats, and complex carbs. These will keep you full for longer and are good for your digestive system. The order of your meals should be complex carbs, then simple carbs, and eventually any delayed gratification foods you may want.

### The One Week Kick-Start Plan for Fat loss and Muscle Growth

One of the ways of starting the intermittent fasting lifestyle plan is by following this one-week plan. There are numerous ways of doing intermittent fasting. Instead of limiting calorie intake, this lifestyle affords you a brief eating window within which you eat all your meals. Therefore, intermittent fasting is not a diet per se, but a healthy lifestyle and way of eating.

One of the most common ways of following this lifestyle is via the 16/8 fasting protocol. This protocol demands that you fast for 16 hours and then have all your meals inside the 8-hour eating window. Plenty of people prefer this protocol because it is much easier to follow. keep in mind that at least 8 hours of this diet include your sleeping time. Therefore, you fast for 8 hours and sleep for an additional 8 hours. Here is a look at the best ways to start this program. While it may sound a little difficult at first, it really is simple once you get used to it. all you need to do is be patient for a while and you will enjoy this lifestyle complete with the body that you will end up in.

# Monday meal program

- First meal: Chia seeds pudding
- Snack: Orange fruit
- Second meal: Fried chicken salad
- Snack: Muesli bar
- Supper: Chicken curry

# Tuesday meal program

- First meal: Whey protein shake
- Snack: Assorted nuts
- Second meal: Vegetarian chickpea salad
- Snack: An apple
- Supper: Quinoa salad

# Wednesday meal program

- First meal: A vanilla whey protein shake
- Snack: A protein bar
- Second meal: Tuna salad sandwiches
- Snack: Yoghurt
- Supper: Fried rice with mixed veggies

# Thursday meal program

- First meal: Fried eggs
- Snack: Banana
- Second meal: Broccoli and carrot salad
- Snack: Almonds and dark chocolate
- Dinner: Chicken garlic

# Friday meal plan

- First meal: coconut chocolate protein balls
- Snack: Scrambled egg
- Second meal: Taco salad
- Snack: Almond nuts

- o   Supper: Chicken salad

## Saturday meal plan

- o   First meal: Paleo breakfast bar
- o   Snack: Hummus carrots
- o   Second meal: Chickpea and avocado salad
- o   Snack: Zucchini chips
- o   Dinner: Chicken and fresh vegetables

## Sunday meal plan

- o   First meal: A protein smoothie
- o   Snack: Mixed nuts
- o   Second meal: Chicken salad
- o   Snack: Whey protein
- o   Supper: Quinoa salad

# Actions for Insane and Rapid Fat Loss

***1. Fast for longer:*** If you want to lose weight very rapidly, then there are a couple of things that you should do. One is to fast regularly. For instance, if you are on the 16-8 fasting protocol, you will fast for 16 hours with an 8-hour eating window. Basically, if you fast for longer, then you will shed more pounds.

*Increase your fast days:* You can increase the frequency of your fasts. For example, the 5-2 protocol requires you to eat normally for five days and then fast for 2 days. Instead of fasting for 2 days, consider increasing this to 3 days. This means that for 3 days a week, you will limit your food intake to a maximum of 500 to 600 calories.

***2. Consider doing fasted cardio:*** One of the best ways of losing body fat is through fasted cardio. This is when you do your cardio workouts as you fast. When you work out on an empty stomach, your body will be forced to tap into fat reserves in the body in order to produce energy. Your body will derive the energy it needs to power your workouts from stored fat reserves.

Therefore, if you want to lose weight rapidly, reduce your caloric intake and work out on an empty stomach in order to burn stored fats. However, approach these tactics with caution because you could feel weak, dizzy, or faint.

# Chapter 8: Maintaining the Fast

It is crucial that intermittent fasting is maintained for the long term. This is the best way for you to benefit from this amazing lifestyle. Maintaining this lifestyle in the long run, requires focus, dedication, and making the right choices. For instance, you need to make sure that you tailor intermittent fasting so that it works for you.

## Make Intermittent Fasting Work for You

There is no single way of making intermittent fasting perfect for everyone. People are different with varying lifestyles and preferences. However, any healthy person can benefit from this lifestyle. This is because it is safe for you and you can practice it as often as you like.

The crucial aspect is to ensure that you are receiving all the nutrition that your body requires. You can choose a particular diet to follow such as the Mediterranean diet or ketogenic diet so as to benefit for the long term.

Try and make intermittent fasting work for you. For instance, if you have to wake up early, need to work the night shift, have a family or spouse and anything of that nature, that your life will still proceed normally even as you adapt the fasting lifestyle. You should also keep trying and experimenting until you find what works for you.

Lastly, you should keep your focus on what you wish to achieve with intermittent fasting. Weight loss is, of course, one of the major benefits but there are numerous other benefits too. They include low blood sugar, lower blood pressure, reduced inflammation, better coronary heart health, and so much more. Focusing on these numerous benefits should motivate you sufficiently to stick with this lifestyle.

## Why You Should Stick with Intermittent Fasting Long-Term

### 1. Effortless fat burning

If you want to lose weight and keep it off in the long run, then your best bet is intermittent fasting. This lifestyle that involves cycles of fasting and eating has been proven over and over again as the best and safest approach to shedding fat, losing weight and keeping it off for the long term.

All other typical diets provide unimpressive results replete with weight regain over time. This can lead to frustrations. Only intermittent fasting lifestyle is able to aid with fat burning that can lead to greater weight loss compared to a typical calorie-restriction diet.

### 2. End Insatiable Hunger

There is often concern raised about hunger throughout the day as dieters fast. Such concerns are not unfounded based on past experiences with other diets. As you fast, your body will enter the fat-burning mode. However, hunger pangs will fade as soon as fatty acids enter your bloodstream. The brain will not place demands on the body for energy if it starts receiving energy from fat-based fuels. As such, you can expect to feel satiated as you fast.

### 3. Sufficient energy for your Entire Day

Even as you fast, you are unlikely to feel hungry or lack energy. The reason for this lack of lethargy is that the body will not be relying on fluctuating carbs stores as a source of energy. Carbs are our regular source of energy but can be unreliable when compared to the fast diet. As we fast, the body gets to receive consistent energy so that the body is fueled and not depleted of energy.

### 4. Intermittent fasting motivates you to make healthy choices

There is sufficient evidence that most dieters who follow intermittent fasting lifestyle tend to stick with it. While this may surprise some, it really is to be expected simply because the benefits are immense. There is a school of thought out there that says our daily willpower is largely limited. This is why people usually give up on ordinary diets that are so restrictive. Intermittent fasting, on the other hand, gives you plenty of leeways to make independent decisions leaving you with an abundant willpower to stick with the lifestyle.

### 5. Increased longevity

Both calorie restriction and intermittent fasting lifestyles have been proven to slow down or stop the onset of disease and boost health span. If you do not have any chronic conditions such as cancer, heart disease, high blood pressure, or diabetes, then your chances of suffering from these conditions are drastically reduced. These are huge benefits of intermittent fasting yet you do not need to suffer calorie restrictions or limited food choice.

# How to Handle Initial Fasting Challenges

*Have the right mindset:* You really need to have the right mindset when you start fasting. If you start to feel hungry just hours into your fast, then you should try and focus on other more crucial matters. You should make sure that you take precautionary measures such as drinking lots of water, drinking coffee or green tea. These will keep your hunger at bay and allow you to continue with your fast. Always keep in mind the reasons why you adopted this lifestyle and the benefits it affords your entire system.

*Learn to discern between psychological and physical hunger:* There is a huge difference between physical and psychological hunger. Physical hunger is easily satisfied by eating a meal or even snacking. This type of hunger is felt gradually and is satiated easily without any guilt feelings. Emotional hunger is rather different. This type of hunger can happen suddenly and may feel urgent. It causes specific cravings and causes you to eat a lot more than you should. When you eat due to psychological hunger, you will feel uncomfortably full and you will feel terribly guilty for your actions.

*Keep your mind and body active:* It is important that you keep as busy as you fast. Keeping busy and focusing on work or other tasks will keep your mind from hunger and food. If you can then you should try and stay occupied. For instance, you should try to immerse yourself in activities that you relish especially during morning hours. You are more productive in the morning so try and stay busy during this period. Keep in mind that even as you fast, you are losing weight and shedding off the unhealthy fats.

***Take a tablespoon or two of Psyllium Husk:*** This is an edible soluble fiber that does your body plenty of good. Psyllium Husk is also a prebiotic and is a common dietary supplement. If you take this product on a regular basis, it will expand and draw water from the colon. It is an efficient colon cleanser and will eliminate waste efficiently. Even as it works on your body, you will not feel any abdominal discomfort such as bloating. Also, Psyllium will promote a healthy heart and positively impact cholesterol levels.

***Overcoming hunger pangs:*** Dieters generally suffer from hunger pangs only for a brief period of time. Most people claim that hunger pangs tend to disappear within a period of two to three weeks. Hunger is barely noticeable beyond the fourth week.

# How to Make Intermittent Fasting Easy on the Body

## 1. Take Water and Beverages to Stay Hydrated

This is one of the simplest tips yet it is mostly avoided by dieters. It is advisable to drink plenty of water throughout the day and remain hydrated. You should also drink other non-caloric beverages. These will not only hydrate you but will help to stave off hunger. Sometimes water may taste a little bland. In such a case, you may add a dash of lemonade. You should not worry about making numerous trips to the bathroom. Water flushes out toxins from the body and keeps you hydrated.

## 2. Drink Bone Broth

Sometimes you may wish to increase your energy levels by taking bone broth. Bone broth contains almost zero calories yet it helps to keep hunger pangs at bay. Research shows that bone broth actually suppresses appetite. It also has anti-obesity properties and does a great job at regulating blood sugar. Take bone broth whenever hunger pangs bother you persistently.

### 3. Consult a nutrition expert

If you want, you may consult a nutritionist and get insights on how to manage the fast. This health expert can expertly guide you and advise you on the changes that you are embarking on. Whenever that you are unsure of something, you should reach out and ask for assistance or advice.

# Tracking Progress and Keeping Motivated

A lot of people start a dieting protocol but then give up shortly thereafter. The reason for this is often because of lack of motivation, little or no progress, and a tough regime or rules and restrictions. Fortunately, this is hardly the case when it comes to intermittent fasting. First, you should accept that intermittent fasting is a lifestyle and not an overnight fast. Losing weight takes a bit of time. Therefore be a little more patient in order to see success eventually.

### *1. Use a mirror to observe your progress*

As soon as you begin this lifestyle, take a look at yourself in the mirror. Observe your body closely and identify the sections that require some work and those where layers of fat need to be worked on. If possible, take photos of yourself then keep observing and noting any changes that occur over time.

### *2. Eat a variety of foods*

Rather than consume one type of food or a small variety, you should consider eating a wider variety of foods. Eating just one food type or a limited variety eventually becomes boring. It is ideal to find out more about the foods that you should eat. These should be unprocessed, healthy, fresh, and whole. Once you discover a variety of foods, you will then be able to enjoy your meals even more.

### 3. Find a suitable partner

You may not know it but working with a partner is highly recommended. This partner could be a spouse, a sibling, or a close friend who shares your passions. You can go through the entire diet and meal plans with this partner and then be each other's coach during workouts. A partner is great to have because you can motivate each other, go shopping together, and generally share this journey with someone close to you.

### 4. Use before and after photos

Photos are crucial because they motivate you. It is often encouraging when you view photos and note how far you have come. Photos are very motivational. Think about the before – after photos in 3, 6, and 9 months. The difference is amazing and the results will definitely impress you and encourage many others.

### 5. Other things you can do

There are a couple of other things that you can do to keep track of progress, observe changes and developments, and stay motivated. Grab some weighing scales and weigh yourself. If you can determine your weight, you should then weight yourself occasionally, probably once every two weeks. Note down measurements each time you measure your weight.

You can also take measurements around your waist, chest, arms, and legs. If you lead a suitable intermittent fasting, then you will notice a reduction in these measurements. For instance, your waist measurements should reduce drastically when you fast. You should also work out regularly. Regular workouts and physical activity help to keep you physically fit and assist with weight loss.

You should also check any skin folds that you have. Skin folds constitute excessive skin which becomes visible due to fat loss around the body. If you follow these simple tips and ideas, then there is no doubt that you will attain your weight loss goals.

# Chapter 9: Diseases Treated or Cured

Fasting has been part of the human culture for centuries. Doctors have advocated the use of fasting for different reasons including treatment and diagnosis of disease. In recent years, intermittent fasting has emerged as a reliable pathway for treating numerous conditions and diseases. There is anecdotal evidence as well as numerous testimonies from individuals who have experienced healing of one disease or another. Some patients have provided credible evidence of chronic conditions getting cured.

## 1. Type II Diabetes

Can intermittent fasting cure type II diabetes? This is very possible. The reason is that intermittent fasting can help to lower your blood sugar levels. These levels can be so low, such that you may not require the use of medication.

This idea of using intermittent fasting to treat diabetes has actually been fronted by a medical doctor and kidney specialist, Dr. Jason Fung. Dr. Fung works as a nephrologist at the Intensive Dietary Management Clinic in Toronto, Canada. In the course of his work, he came across numerous patients suffering from diabetes and kidney failure.

He has been using intermittent fasting to help treat diabetes in his patients with excellent outcomes. Apparently, type II diabetes is the most common form of diabetes and accounts to 80% - 90% of cases. It is associated with obesity, unhealthy eating, and usually manifests later in life.

A major aspect of diabetes is insulin resistance. The body usually produces the hormone insulin in order to regulate blood sugar. Insulin facilitates the transfer of glucose in the blood into the cells for use as energy. However, for some unexplained reasons, body tissues are sometimes unresponsive to insulin such that there is too much glucose in the blood.

Patients are normally put on medication that helps to direct glucose into the cells. However, according to Dr. Fung, this is the wrong approach. Intermittent fasting can help to regulate blood sugar and effectively help to treat type II diabetes. When you fast, the body is able to burn off the excess sugar which causes the cells and tissues to become responsive to insulin once more.

Type II diabetes is an entire reversible condition according to Dr. Fung. By fasting regularly, patients tend to lose weight and insulin resistance is overcome. In many instances, patients even stop taking medication.

## 2. Alzheimer's and Parkinson's Diseases

We have already heard about the power of intermittent fasting and how to can cleanse the body and improve health. However, it has been established that intermittent fasting is able to positively affect certain neurodegenerative diseases like Parkinson's and Alzheimer's.

There is concrete evidence, according to a study by Dr. Mark Mattson of the John Hopkins School of Medicine. The study reveals that intermittent fasting causes the brain to perform in much healthier ways. According to his research findings, fasting a couple of times each week enhances neural connections in a part of the brain known as the hippocampus.

*How this helps with neurodegenerative diseases*

According to research findings, Dr. Mattson believes that fasting challenges the brain. In response, the brain activates certain stress responses known as adaptive stress responses. These help the brain to cope with the disease. When viewed from an evolutionary perspective, it makes good sense why the brain should be responding so well even when you have had any nourishment for hours.

Fasting turns fat into ketones to produce energy. The process encourages a healthy transformation in the region of the brain that is crucial for memory and learning and overall brain health. This actually works and scientists are excited. Burning fat to produce ketones helps the brain to transform in response to stress. The same thing occurs when we exercise. Dr. Mattson advises patients to attempt two different of performing intermittent fasting. These are the 5:2 protocol and the time-restricted protocol. Dr. Matt also advises some regular physical activity. Exercising is a requirement for this fasting-inspired healing approach.

## 3. Multiple Sclerosis

In patients suffering from multiple sclerosis, their immune system will wrongfully attack links that attach nerve cells together and prevents them from properly communicating. The immune system not only attacks the nerve links but also causes them harm. This results in undesirable outcomes such as chronic pain, muscle weakness, coordination problems, and fatigue.

Unfortunately, there is currently no cure for multiple sclerosis victims. Current treatment options available to patients only help to manage symptoms. There have been suggestions that dietary interventions could help the body battle this condition.

Researchers from the Washington University School of Medicine in St Louis, MO, believe that interventions such as following the intermittent fasting protocol can help in the management of this condition. One of the research scientists involved in this study, Dr. Laura Piccio says that there is anecdotal evidence about patients who have regained the ability to walk after starting the intermittent fasting lifestyle. However, the doctor claims that this fasting lifestyle greatly helps with the management of symptoms of multiple sclerosis. This makes a huge difference in the lives of patients who live with this chronic condition.

The researchers first conducted tests in the lab with mice models and obtained impressive results. They then tried intermittent fasting on human beings and the outcomes were absolutely phenomenal. The results of the study have been published in the Cell Metabolism journal.

## 4. High Blood Pressure

Fasting has huge benefits for your heart health and consequently high blood pressure. According to cardiologist Dr. Ahmed, MD, fasting for short periods of time on a regular basis has numerous advantages to the body and generally to your health. It basically pays to limit your calorie intake.

When you fast, you generally lose weight. Weight loss leads to less work for the heart. Fasting also stresses the body sufficiently in a positive manner. The heart becomes stronger and no longer struggles to pump blood.

Research on health benefits of intermittent fasting was published in Nutrition and Healthy Aging journal in June 2018. The findings of the research show that intermittent fasting helps you lose weight and lowers blood pressure. The study focused on obese individuals and they all lost substantial amounts of weight. Plenty of other crucial markers also indicated remarkable improvements.

These include cholesterol, insulin resistance, and fat mass. They all decreased remarkably which in return support the reduction in high blood pressure. The researchers support the 16/8 protocol which supports impressive blood pressure reduction.

## 5. Heart and Cardiovascular Diseases

Some of the major causes of heart and cardio diseases include excessive body weight, high cholesterol levels, diabetes, and high blood pressure. Researchers have shown that intermittent fasting or restricting food and drink can significantly improve risk factors related to the heart and cardiovascular system.

One study shows that individuals who follow the intermittent fasting lifestyle have better heart health than those who do not follow such a lifestyle. If you lose weight because of intermittent fasting and shed off fat, then your coronary health and cardiovascular system will be in much better shape.

Also, intermittent fasting couples with an active lifestyle will lead to lower blood sugar. It also reduces your levels of low-density lipoproteins sometimes referred to as bad cholesterol.

## 6. Brain Health

Intermittent fasting has been shown to reduce inflammation throughout the body. It is also an excellent weight loss tool and great for supercharging the brain. Most chronic diseases that we face are as a result of inflammation. These include diabetes, dementia, Alzheimer's, and so on.

Intermittent fasting reduces inflammation through autophagy, ketones, and insulin management. Also, when we fast, more brain cells are created. According to Dr. Mark Mattson of John Hopkins University, fasting has been shown to rapidly increase neurogenesis in the brain. The term neurogenesis refers to the creation or development of new brain cells and related nerve tissues. Fasting also boosts the production of a protein known simply as BDNF which is a miraculous growth protein. This protein helps the brain to grow, change, and adapt to new and changing environments.

## 7. Cancer

Intermittent fasting is mostly used to boost weight loss. However, it is known to have numerous other benefits ranging from brain health to protection against diseases such as diabetes. Patients suffering from different types of cancers will benefit immensely by adopting an intermittent fasting lifestyle.

There is widely accepted evidence that that fasting, especially intermittent fasting slows and hinders the growth of cancerous tumors. Intermittent fasting also reduces treatment side effects, supports chemotherapy treatment making it more effective, prevents recurrences, and drastically increases survival rates of patients.

While there is still a lot of research going on, current verifiable information shows that intermittent fasting helps to fight cancer, reduces chances for any new cancer cells and supports healing including enhancing chemotherapy and other treatment options. Fasting also denies cancer tumors the nutrition they need to grow and thrive.

## 8. Gut Health

Intermittent fasting is beneficial for your gut. It promotes gut health in different ways. The human gut contains a myriad of microbes that include fungi, viruses, and bacteria of all sizes and shapes. There are over a thousand species of these microbes in your gut and they greatly affect and impact your health.

Gut microbiota can alter the way the body metabolizes food. They even let the brain known when we are hungry and when we are full. It is now evident that fasting has a huge effect on gut microbiota. By fasting and improving the quality of nutrients, we positively affect gut microbiota.

The body has for thousands of years been used to fasting and being calorie free. It is only in recent years that we had access to food on a 24-hour basis, 7 days a week. By cutting back on nutrition, the digestive system takes a break and the gut bacteria take a break. The quality of gut microbial and their nature improves remarkably when we fast. You can find out a lot more information about this by following this link. Food scarcity is really what our bodies had been used to. We thrive when there is a temporary shortage. The stress caused by fasting helps the body to perform at optimum levels.

## 9. Autoimmune Disease

There are research studies that have shown potential benefits of intermittent fasting for autoimmune diseases such as rheumatoid arthritis and fibromyalgia. This lifestyle is also very promising when it comes to other autoimmune diseases like multiple sclerosis, lupus, and so on.

Basically, when you fast for an extended period of time, the body gets an opportunity to relax and rest. Your body takes this opportunity to heal, recover, and repair because it is not busy digesting food or protecting against inflammatory substances in the food we eat.

When it heals, a lot of positive things happen. For instance, it repairs a leaky gut which is the precursor to all autoimmune diseases. A leaky gut is a term that refers to intestinal permeability. When leaks are sealed in the lining of the intestines, the symptoms of autoimmune diseases can then be managed.

## 10. Obesity and Overweight

Intermittent fasting has been acknowledged by numerous dieters as an effective weight loss tool. In fact, most people who follow this simple lifestyle do so in order to lose weight and keep it off. The reason why intermittent fasting is so popular as a weight loss tool is because it does not involve extreme effort, constant hunger, or calorie counting.

There are a number of studies out that show this to be factual. A test was done where obese individuals structured their meals such that they fasted for a total of 16 hours per day but were allowed to eat anything they wanted in the next 8 hours. The results were impressive and showed how these individuals lost some modest weight.

Now the same group of obese individuals was requested to go without food for 16 hours but then could only eat 350 less calories during the eating window. This study was conducted by Krista Varady, an associate professor of nutrition at the University of Illinois in Chicago. The participants all lost significant amounts of weight. If done correctly and coupled with regular workouts, intermittent fasting will enable overweight and obese persons to lose weight and keep it off.

# Chapter 10: Myths, Common Questions, and Considerations for Men and Women

There are numerous benefits that come out of this lifestyle. There are plenty of testimonies as well as anecdotal evidence about people who've lost vast amounts of weight or had a serious condition healed. If you want to enjoy the benefits of intermittent fasting, then you ought to do it correctly. What you need to be able to do is avoid making common mistakes and debunk any myths out there.

## Breakfast Myths

For a long time, we grew up believing that breakfast is the most crucial meal of the day. We were advised to never leave the house without having breakfast. However, the question is, is breakfast really the most important meal of the day? Is it advisable to kick-start the day with a full breakfast meal?

### Myth 1: Breakfast is crucial and is a healthy option

For a long time, we have believed that breakfast is a crucial morning meal and that you had to have breakfast in order to have a great morning. However, this may not necessarily be true. Not all breakfast meals are equal and some options could be unhealthy. The healthiest breakfast should include a protein, whole grain, 100% fruit juice or a fruit.

## Myth 2: Skipping breakfast helps with weight loss

While skipping some meals and cutting back on calories is a great idea, in some instances, it really isn't. Some healthcare experts believe that skipping breakfast can be detrimental to your health in some instances. Hunger may cause you to overindulge later on. You should stick to eating a balanced diet always.

## Myth 3: Breakfast is the most crucial meal of the day

We have for a long time believed that breakfast is the most important meal of the day. However, the truth is that there is no single meal that is the most important of the day. The crucial aspect to consider on any meal is the quality and quantity consumed at each meal.

# 10 Popular Questions on Intermittent Fasting

## Question 1: What is intermittent fasting?

Intermittent fasting is an eating pattern where you cycle between the period of eating and fasting. It is not a diet that tells you to eat one type of food and not eat another food type. However, it is a lifestyle where you fast for a couple of hours, usually 16 hours per day and then have your meals in the remaining time period.

## Question 2: What are the benefits of this lifestyle?

Intermittent fasting has numerous benefits. Most people follow this lifestyle in order to lose weight and keep it off. With intermittent lifestyle, you lose weight gradually which means you lose it possibly for good and instead strong, lean muscle.

You can expect increased life expectancy. Studies at the National Institute of Ageing show that animals tend to age slower and live longer if they eat fewer calories. You will notice an improvement in your hormone performance. For instance, you can expect reduced insulin levels, an increase in HGH or human growth hormone, and a reduction in blood sugar levels.

These all support weight loss, lower risk of heart disease and diabetes, and for maintaining lean muscle mass. Intermittent fasting promotes a healthy body by eliminating inflammation in the body.

### 4. Why and how does intermittent fasting burn fat?

When you limit your calorie intake, there is less glucose on the body. This signals the body to rely more on stored fats than from glucose derived from carbs in your diet. Since the body needs energy to function, it will reach into stored fats and start burning them in order to produce the energy it needs.

### 5. What makes it so effective?

One of the reasons why intermittent fasting is so powerful is mostly due to the adaptive response from cells. The response results in a reduction in inflammation and oxidative stress. The body also improves cellular production and optimizes the body's metabolism. Intermittent fasting helps the body to handle stress much better especially when cells have to cope with nutrition limitations.

### 6. What types of intermittent fasting protocols are out there?

There are many ways of doing intermittent fasting. There are different protocols that you can follow. We have 5-2 protocol, the 16/8 protocol, and the alternate day fasting protocol. There is also the 24-hour fast that you can do probably twice or more times per month. There is generally no one protocol that is better than the other. It is simply advisable that you identify one that works for you and stick by it.

### 7. Where do I begin?

Once you determine that you wish to pursue this kind of lifestyle, you should then think and plan how to begin the journey. Plan to begin fasting on a particular day. It could be a Monday or any other day of the week. The night just before you begin is your first night before intermittent fasting. Ensure that you eat a meal loaded with protein, complex carbs, and vegetables. Complex carbs and proteins will keep you feeling full for much longer. When you wake up in the morning, you will already have fasted for eight hours. At this point, you should go about your business as usual. Take coffee, black tea, or even water should you start feeling hungry again.

### 8. How do I do intermittent fasting for weight loss?

According to experts, the simplest way to lose weight with an intermittent fasting lifestyle is to fast once per week. Ideally, we lose weight when we consume fewer calories than we burn. One-day fast means once you have your evening meal, you will then eat nothing for the rest of the time until the following day's dinner. As you fast, your body will rely on stored fat to generate energy.

### 9. What foods are best after breaking the fast?

Quality nutrition is crucial if you want to enjoy the benefits of fasting. If you end your fast around dinner time, then you should have your dinner right there and then. However, if you end your fast around four in the afternoon, then you should have a snack as you wait for dinner.

Whatever meal you decide to have, just ensure that it contains sufficient amounts of assorted vegetables, high-quality proteins such as chicken or fish, a carbohydrate like brown rice, sweet potato and so on. Most dieters usually eat clean after a fast. This is highly advisable because healthy eating results in healthy individuals.

### 10. Can I exercise during my fasting window?

You may sometimes wish to train in a fasted state. This is likely to result in significant weight loss. Fasted training or fasted cardio is quite popular especially with individuals who wish to lose a lot of weight within a short period of time.

On other non-fast days, you can engage in more rigorous workouts. You can go for jogging or even a hill run. Work on your muscle and develop them so that you are both healthy and fit. Always be careful and watch your energy levels before working out.

# Specifically Men and Intermittent Fasting – Things to Consider

*1. Stubborn belly fat*: A lot of men carry a pot belly which never seems to go away no matter how hard they work out. Fortunately, intermittent fasting offers you the best solution yet. By following this lifestyle, you are likely to lose the belly fat and have a flat tummy again. Developing abdominal muscles is also possible

*2. Human growth hormone:* As you fast, your body produces higher amounts of HGH. This is an absolutely important hormone that supports growth and development of tissue and muscles. Higher levels of HGH are necessary to keep you looking great and to slow down aging.

*3. Develop strong*, *lean muscle:* Intermittent fasting helps you lose fat and shed pounds. This also presents an excellent opportunity to develop muscles. Anaerobic workouts are crucial if you are to develop a strong body with lean muscles throughout.

You will, therefore, need to work out regularly, eat the right kinds of foods, and fast occasionally.

**4. *Improve your fitness level***: As you fast, you should also maintain your fitness levels. It is advisable to work out regularly and live an active lifestyle. If you work out regularly then you will become physically fit and strong. Your challenge will be to maintain this level of fitness for the long term.

**5. *Eat smaller portions***: You are probably used to eating fairly large food portions both at home and whenever you eat at a restaurant. These large portions are no good for you. They simply help you to pile up the kilos. Learn to reduce the size of your portions so that you consume only the calories that your body needs.

# Specifically Women and Intermittent Fasting – Things to Consider

**1. *Weight loss***: You have probably tried just about all diets out there in order to lose weight and keep it off. Fortunately, there is intermittent fasting. This healthy lifestyle will ensure that you lose weight if done correctly. There are ways of speeding up weight loss. These include doing cardio exercises in a fasted state and fasting for longer periods.

**2. *Stubborn belly fat***: Just like men women sometimes also struggle with stubborn belly fat. If you work out regularly and reduce your calorie intake, then you will slowly but surely lose fat around your abdomen area and keep it off. Make sure that you follow your preferred fasting protocol as required.

**3. *Fasting and hormones***: One of the major differences between males and females when it comes to fasting is how much they are affected by hormones. According to scientists, women's hormones are affected by fasting much more compared to men.

They believe this is because of a protein known as kisspeptin. Fortunately, intermittent fasting can help in the regulation of hormones. When you fast, work out, and eat healthily, your body will better regulate hormones.

**4. Hunger cues**: Once you begin fasting, you are likely to experience plenty of hunger. A lot of the appetite hormones occur in higher levels in women than in men. Try not to ignore hunger cues. Instead, prepare well for your fasting session by eating well the night before. Increase your protein intake, drink lots of water. Also, fast maybe once or twice a week and on non-consecutive days.

**5. Consider crescendo fasting**: This is a fasting protocol developed specifically for women. This fasting approach is kinder to the body and will help your hormones to settle down and not bother you that much. There are definite benefits to crescendo fasting. For instance, you can expect to see your energy levels increase, lose both body weight and body fat, and experience almost no hormonal challenges.

# Chapter 11: Popular Intermittent Fasting Celebrities

Intermittent fasting lifestyle has definitely caught the attention of people around the world. Celebrities have not been left out. Everybody has heard how awesome this lifestyle is and how impressive the results are. This is why a lot of people, including celebrities, are joining the bandwagon.

There have been many diets that made headlines in the past couple of decades. These include the grapefruit diet, the low-fat diet, and even the Master Cleanse. Sadly, they did not last for long. However, intermittent fasting is different because it is not a diet but more of a lifestyle and way of eating. It involves periods of fasting and eating. Most celebrities have endorsed one or two protocols even though there are more than five common ones. Here are some of the celebrities who have chosen the intermittent fasting lifestyle.

## 1. Jennifer Lopez

One of the best-known celebrities who practices intermittent fasting is Jennifer Lopez, also known as J. Lo. While she is always glamorous, J. Lo works extremely hard to look the way she does. Part of her lifestyle involves not eating anything for a period of eight hours per day. She also works out regularly and eats healthy. This shows how well she takes care of her body and overall health.

## 2. Nicole Kidman

This Australian actress is also said to be an avid follower of this lifestyle. Like J. Lo, Nicole Kidman prefers to follow the 8-hour fasting rule. She prefers to fast regularly and when she eventually sits down to eat she opts for veggies and lean protein.

### 3. Justin Theroux

Justin is not just a popular celebrity but is also conscious about his health. This is why his trainer convinced him to follow the intermittent fasting lifestyle. Since he discovered this lifestyle, Justin has been fasting for 12 hours between 7.00 pm and 7.00 am and eats only outside of these hours.

### 4. Beyoncé

One of the leading female artists of all time is Beyoncé Carter. Beyoncé, or Bey as she is popularly known, has been following this lifestyle for a couple of years now. While she has never confirmed it, numerous outlets have confirmed that she does. Beyoncé looks great, is superbly fit, and seems not to age. All these can probably be attributed to intermittent fasting.

### 5. Terry Crews

Terry was among the very first celebrities to come out and proclaim his love for this lifestyle. He also follows it religiously. His first meal each day is at 2.00 pm. His eating window, which is only 8 hours long, stretches to 10.00 pm. He fasts every single day for 16 hours but enjoys a cup of coffee or tea as he fasts. Apart from fasting, he also works out regularly and has developed some serious muscles.

### 6. Hugh Jackman

We all love Hugh Jackman and his excellent acting skills. He was also among the very first celebrities to come out in support of intermittent fasting. like Terry Crews, he too prefers to fast for 16 hours during his fasting days and then has all his meals in the 8-hour eating window.

### 7. Antoni Porowski

Even Antoni is an ardent intermittent fasting adherent. While he does not flaunt this lifestyle, he is keen on maintaining his health and fitness. He usually has his first meal at around 12.00 noon and then keeps this eating window open until 8.00 pm in the evening. He then eats nothing until noon the following day. His amazing good looks, lean physique, and easy going nature highlight all the aspects of intermittent fasting.

### *Other celebrities*
There are plenty of other celebrities who follow this fasting lifestyle. They include Liv Tyler, Miranda Kerr, and Ben Affleck. After becoming aware of the numerous benefits of intermittent fasting, they all chose to pursue it.

A lot of these celebrities prefer to follow the fast diet where they fast for 2 days and then eat normally for 5 days. They find this protocol easier to follow and gentle on the body. Many celebrities were made aware of this lifestyle through a TV documentary. They love this particular lifestyle because it actually works and results are very visible. Intermittent fasting has also been tried successfully and proven to work effectively.

Others who have chosen to pursue this lifestyle include Fiona Becket of the Guardian and Kate Middleton's uncle. They are both of the opinion that this lifestyle has made a huge impact on other people's lives and they too would love to enjoy similar benefits.

# Conclusion

Intermittent fasting provides one of the most effective lifestyle changes known to man. Those who have turned to this lifestyle have seen such amazing changes and continue to enjoy such a good quality of life. It is why many concede the switch to this lifestyle as the best decision they have ever made in their lives.

This lifestyle is very simple indeed. Unlike other diets and eating fads, it places no demands on its followers other than the requirement to fast for a period of time and then eat during a brief eating window. Such simple requirements have surprisingly great outcomes.

Starting out is really simple. Your first step is to simply understand all about this lifestyle, how it works, and all its benefits. Once you understand and accept the theory aspect, you will then need to start applying it. The transition is absolutely simple. Once you are able to make the transition, you will be able to indulge in this lifestyle and overcome all initial challenges.

It is even easier to follow this lifestyle because there are numerous protocols to choose from. You will not be compelled to follow a particular protocol but will be free to choose the method that you like. The lifestyle is also accommodating and this allows you to make certain changes so that this fasting program suits your lifestyle. And should you make mistakes along the way, you should not despair and give up. Mistakes are part and parcel of the learning process. Simply shake off the dust and start again.

The benefits of intermittent lifestyle are numerous. Intermittent fasting enables you to lose weight and keep it off. It promotes a healthy body by minimizing inflammation. Intermittent fasting helps to cure diseases and treat certain conditions so that you eventually get to enjoy optimum health. If you encounter difficulties, then you should find a reliable individual to consult with. For instance, find a book to read, a website, or an experienced person and talk to them. It is also great if you can find someone to partner with in this journey. Identify a friend, a spouse or close family member and work together. It is always easier when you have someone to encourage and support you along the way.

Motivation: If you need inspiration or motivation, then consider joining a group of individuals who share the same interest. There are plenty of groups across different social media. Find a group, engage members, and share your experiences and challenges. You are bound to find a willing partner, listening ear, and helpful advice. The benefits of this lifestyle are numerous and you should share in these benefits. Remember to drink plenty of water as you fast and exercise on a regular basis. You are bound to succeed if you pursue this lifestyle correctly and adhere to it diligently. Take photos at different stages and note the amazing changes taking place as you follow this amazing lifestyle.

If you enjoyed this book, please leave me a positive review on Amazon as it keeps me being able to produce quality books. Thank you

www.ingramcontent.com/pod-product-compliance
Lightning Source LLC
Chambersburg PA
CBHW072152020426
42334CB00018B/1969